The Hook Up Handbook

28 Fundamentals to Keep Her Coming Back for More

David Perrotta
www.PostGradCasanova.com

Disclaimer

All attempts have been made to verify the information in this book; however, neither the author nor the publisher assumes any responsibility for errors, omissions, or contrary interpretations of the content within.

This book is for entertainment purposes only, and so the views of the author should not be taken as expert instruction or commands. The reader is responsible for his or her own actions.

Neither the author nor the publisher assumes any responsibility or liability on behalf of the purchaser or reader of this book.

Buyer Bonus

As a way of saying thank you for your purchase, I'm offering a FREE video series that's exclusive to my book and blog readers.

It features 3 in-depth videos, where I walk you through how to flirt with girls and avoid debilitating conversation mistakes.

Inside you will learn:

- The 5 conversation mistakes that put you in the friendzone (and how to avoid them).

- My secret conversation framework for flirting with any girl.

- The "invisible trigger" that activates attraction in a woman's mind, often within seconds of meeting you

- A simple way to overcome the 3 "dating roadblocks" that hold 99% of men back from meeting the women they truly want.

...and much, much more.

Download it here:
bit.ly/handbookcourse

Contents

Introduction

What Life Will Look Like When You're Great at Sex...

Do you know how to have the sort of mind-blowing, orgasmic sex that women tell their friends about?

Or do your sex sessions fizzle out in a few minutes and end with a dud?

For most guys, it's the latter. They don't know how to fuck a girl the right way. It's no wonder why so many relationships are in turmoil and so many women cheat.

To be frank, these women want some good sex, and their man just isn't delivering.

If you don't give your woman good sex – whether she's a girlfriend, fuck buddy, or wife – she's not going to stick around for long. And if by chance she does, she'll probably get some on the side (even if you think she's a "good girl" who would never do a thing like that).

On the other hand, here are some things you can expect when you know how to have great sex with women:

- You'll enjoy the sex a lot more yourself and actually look forward to it instead of being insecure about it.

- Women will literally get hooked on sex with you – they'll want to keep coming back again and again.

- It'll be a lot easier to get a girlfriend and make her want you.

- Your girlfriend/wife will be a lot less likely to "get some" on the side.

- Your sex reputation will spread, especially if you're in a small social circle (and other women will get curious about you and want to see for themselves).

- You'll be a lot more confident when flirting with women, because you'll know you can give her a great experience in bed if it comes to that (whereas if you're insecure about your sexual prowess, you'll likely sabotage your chances with women to stop the possibility of sex happening).

(If none of those bullet points above sound familiar, then you're probably not great at sex just yet.)

So yeah, sex is pretty damn important. If you want to have fulfilling relationships with women, you need to get good in the sack. This book is going to help you do it.

And even if you are great at sex, there's always room for improvement. That way, you can keep yourself sharp and your women satisfied.

As you build your sexual prowess and ability, you will see the world in a different light. You'll look at women differently, and they'll see you differently as a result.

You'll give off a different vibe and energy... One of confidence and sexual understanding.

Women will sense this vibe more and more as you continue to improve, and you'll become a naturally attractive man.

I've seen it happen in my life over the years, as well as in the lives of many of my friends.

And if you read through this entire book and apply what you learn, it will happen to you as well.

You'll become the guy who goes for what he wants with women.

You'll be the guy who has women moaning from his bedroom every night. And you'll be the guy who women rave about to their friends.

It doesn't matter whether you have a lot of sexual experience or none at all...

The sex fundamentals you're about to learn will work for you. And while all women are different, they all respond to the same fundamentals.

So sit down and buckle up. The way you have sex is about to change forever.

Who Am I to Write a Book About Sex?

Before we go any further, you might be thinking, "Who is this guy, and what does he know about great sex?!"

I get it, man. You've been fed shitty sex advice for years, by "scientists" who probably haven't had sex in decades and nerds who are probably still virgins.

(I read all their books and listened to their audiobooks while I was doing research, and I cringed the whole time...)

You're not about to trust your sex life to another random schmuck (or sexless nerd) who doesn't know what the hell he's talking about (or hasn't *been there* and *done that*).

So let me introduce myself. My name is Dave Perrotta. I'm a dating coach, best-selling author, and the founder of PostGradCasanova.

And while I can rant about how I've sold tens of thousands of books and had sex with hundreds of women from all over the world—or how my blog gets over 150,000 visits per month—I don't want to be a douche.

But I haven't always been able to give women orgasm after orgasm.

Things used to be A LOT different...

Hell, the first few girls I kissed remarked that I was "one hell of a bad kisser."

In fact, I was so bad that I accidentally gave one of them a fat lip... from kissing! Talk about awkward...

(And no, she never talked to me again... and I'm pretty sure she's a lesbian now!)

And when I eventually started having sex, things didn't get much better.

I still remember one cringeworthy sexual experience from back then...

***

My friend and I had just brought two girls back to their college dorm. We'd met them at a party an hour or so beforehand, and it was ON. We all knew what was going to go down that night...

We walked into their dorm room and noticed their beds were only separated by a few feet. We gave each other a devious glance – we knew what was in store...

After a quick drink and some flirting, we started

hooking up with the girls.

Clothes came off. I started having sex with my girl, and he started having sex with his.

(It was a bit funny to see out of the corner of my eye – he was a 6'5'' dude from the college football team, and his girl was about 5'1.)

All was going well…

Until a couple minutes in…

I was trying to hold it back, but I lost control…

Boom. I came after less than five minutes.

"What happened? Are you all good?" she asked.

"Yeah, I just came… I usually don't finish this quickly…" I shrugged.

"Oh, okay…" she said.

But my friend was far from finished…

As my girl and I sat there on the bed, he kept fucking and making his girl moan for an hour.

I felt awkward, inadequate, and embarrassed. It's bad enough when you finish in less than 5 minutes… but it's even worse when your friend is clearly giving the other girl an amazing sexual experience just a few feet away.

***

How I Learned to Be Great at Sex

In the early days, my sex life had a lot of mediocre and embarrassing moments.

I couldn't last very long, and I didn't really know what the hell I was doing *even when I could* manage to last longer than a few minutes.

I always felt apprehensive when I brought a girl home, because I wasn't confident I could give her a great experience.

I knew I had to do something about this problem...

After some careful thought, it seemed like there were two big things I needed to do...

The first? Talk to guys who were great at sex and learn what they were doing in the bedroom.

The second? Get more sexual experience with women so I could learn what different girls like, train myself to last longer, and gain more sexual confidence.

I knew the second wouldn't be too difficult. My conversation and flirting skills were improving rapidly, and I had no issue picking up women and bringing them to the bedroom.

*(If you have trouble flirting and talking to women, I recommend checking out my free video course on conversation and flirting at: **bit.ly/handbookcourse**.)*

The first would be a little tougher. It'd require me to open myself up and admit that I wasn't where I wanted to be in my sex life. But I had no choice.

So I approached a few of the guys in my fraternity who I knew were great at sex…

These guys had a reputation. You'd always hear women moaning from their bedrooms, and the girls on campus would gossip about it. They all wanted to experience their bedroom prowess and see what the hype was about.

A few of the guys laughed at first, but I think they appreciated my honesty because they started to reveal their secrets…

(Which, to my surprise, were actually quite simple…)

I started applying a few of these secrets with the girls I had sex with, and I noticed an immediate improvement.

I still wasn't quite where I wanted to be, but I was getting better quickly.

As I applied these secrets with more and more women, I began to build on them and experiment with new things. Some of them worked, and some of them didn't. So I took what worked and kept moving forward.

***

Fast-forward seven years. I've lived in seven different countries and slept with hundreds more women, and I've continued to improve in the bedroom."

I've learned something new from practically all of these women... from what they like and don't like, to what I can do better, to what women really need and crave, and a lot more.

I've also learned to last as long as I want (or, as long as the girl can take it!) and give women mind-blowing orgasms. I now enjoy sex A LOT more too.

My confidence is through the roof because I know I can give any girl an amazing night of sex. This is a stark contrast from my early days, when I just hoped I'd be able to last ten minutes!

I have a lot more confidence when I'm dating women, too. I know I can satisfy a girlfriend in the bedroom, and she won't have the desire to mess around with other guys.

I've also started PostGradCasanova, where I've helped thousands of men improve their confidence, master conversation skills, and have amazing sex lives.

And now, I want to help you.

As I said before, I did a lot of research on the subject of sex, and I was disappointed with what I found. Nerds, virgins, and sexless scientists spouting bullshit.

There are no guys who actually get laid writing about sex. It's time to change that.

I've seen the importance of great sex when it comes to cultivating a strong connection with a woman, and I want to help guys make those deeper connections.

You see, to give a woman great orgasmic sex you don't need to have a gigantic penis, last for hours, or memorize all the special Kamasutra techniques. It's a lot simpler and easier than that.

I've distilled great sex down to a set of fundamentals. I'll show you how to learn, internalize, and apply these fundamentals, so that women will literally crave sex with you (and have orgasm after orgasm).

This book will reshape the way you think about sex, and your future women will thank you for reading it.

How The Hook Up Handbook Will Help You...

This book is divided into 7 key parts:

I. The Sexual Landscape (why most men are mediocre in the bedroom, how women think about sex, and what really makes a woman orgasm)

II. Developing Your Sexy Vibe (become a sexy man and master the right sexual mindsets)

III. The "Setup" Fundamentals (make the first move and master the "build-up" to sex)

IV. The "Foreplay" Fundamentals (get her excited through sexy foreplay, and understand her parts and what to do with them)

V. The Sex Fundamentals (the most pleasurable sex positions; how to be dominant, add variety, infuse passion, build your stamina, use dirty talk, and have orgasmic anal sex)

VI. The Performance Fundamentals (how to last longer in bed, beat performance anxiety, and immerse yourself in the experience)

VII. What to Do After Sex (how to show her you care, and how to guarantee that you see her again)

Part I will help you understand how sex works and how women perceive it.

Part II will help you become a sexy man who radiates sexuality and turns women on from his mere presence.

Part III will help you become a man who makes the first move and has sex with the women he wants.

Part IV will give you the tools you need to get her excited beforehand, so she practically begs you for sex.

Part V will reveal the secrets you need to give her the best sex she's ever had... every time.

Part VI will help you crush performance anxiety so you consistently have great sex (without worrying about how long you'll last).

Part VII will help you make her feel comfortable after sex, so you can further build the connection and see her in the future.

Now it's time to dive into Part I: The Sexual Landscape. So roll your sleeves up and get ready!

How to Use This Book

Anyone can pick up this book and read it – but not everyone will see results.

To get the most out of this book, you must do 2 things:

1. Be open to accepting new ideas.

2. Make an effort to apply the fundamentals.

Sex is a sensitive subject for a lot of guys. Their egos are attached to their sexual ability, so to admit they need help in this area can be a tough blow.

I know, because I had to deal with that tough blow to the ego, too. But I'm glad I did.

Now, if you're not having the quality of sex you want with the type of women you desire, then your sex life could use some improvement.

In this book, you'll learn a set of fundamentals that will help you make that improvement in a big way.

But you can't just read a book like this and expect to get results. You have to actually try and apply the fundamentals in your life – and in the bedroom as well.

Some of these fundamentals will push you out of your comfort zone a bit. But once you try them, you'll see exactly why they drive women so wild.

If you actually apply these fundamentals and master them, you'll attract more women, have an unbelievable sex life, and significantly improve your current and future relationships with women.

Keep this in mind as we go through the book!

Part I:
The Sexual
Landscape

Why Most Men Are Mediocre in the Bedroom

Women have been unsatisfied in the bedroom for centuries.

But here's the crazy part: usually, their men don't even realize it.

According to a survey from HealthyWoman.org [1] 62 percent of women admitted to not being satisfied with their sex lives.

What's more, 79 percent of men *think* their wives are happy or very happy with their sex lives, while only 60 percent of those women say they actually are [1].

So there's a big disconnect here. Men think they're doing at least an "okay" job, when really their women are craving much more.

And from talking to countless women about this (and seeing the relief and satisfaction on their faces after a great session of sex), I can attest to these stats. Hell, I would even say women are far more dissatisfied than the surveys say.

So, what's going on here? Why are women not getting the kind of sex they need?

It comes down to one big reason...

Most men are mediocre in the bedroom!

Sure, they can perform okay from time to time – and even have a great night of sex on rare occasion – but they're not consistent.

I was very inconsistent just a few years ago. Sometimes I'd last 30 minutes and give a girl multiple orgasms, and sometimes I'd struggle to last 5 minutes. Maybe you can relate.

Whatever the case, it's no big surprise that most men are mediocre in the bedroom.

Think about it: As men, we're never really taught how to fuck a girl the right way. There's no introductory class in school between algebra and history titled "Intercourse 101." There's no "how-to" guide that gives a man instructions to please any and every woman he comes into contact with.

As a man, you are left with your dick in your hands, given an infinite amount of Internet porn, and expected to come out on the other side with the knowledge of how to fuck a girl.

And then, if you don't perform well, you feel sexual shame, anxiety, and outright embarrassment. The hard truth is that you might even feel like less of a man. Girls will giggle at you, and the whole sexual experience will become awkward and uncomfortable.

To sum it up, here are a few big reasons why most men are mediocre in the bedroom:

- **They don't last long enough.** It's not about lasting a certain amount of time so much as it is about controlling your own orgasm and finishing whenever you want. This requires good physical stamina as well as the psychological knowledge of how to control the orgasm.

- **They don't know what to do.** They don't know the right way to fuck a girl. Positions, mindsets, the emotional level, etc. — it's all foreign to these guys. They thrust in and out and hope for the best.

- **The skip out on foreplay or do it poorly.** They fail to build up and get the girl excited about the sexual experience. This takes away from the actual intercourse and makes the woman feel unappreciated.

- **They focus only on the girl's pleasure and don't pay themselves any mind (or vice versa).** This one is a bit counterintuitive. When you focus completely on the girl's pleasure, you can get insecure about whether or not she's enjoying the experience, and you can also sacrifice a lot of your own enjoyment.

But if you focus only on your own pleasure, you may end up ignoring her needs and desires, and you also might get overwhelmed and finish prematurely. The key is to pay mind to both your pleasure *and* her pleasure but focus mainly on enjoying and immersing yourself in the overall experience (don't worry, you'll be well equipped to do this by the end of the book).

- They lack variety. They fuck a girl the same way (or a very similar way) just about every time and hardly ever switch it up. The sex gets boring over time.

- They don't infuse the sex with emotion. They focus solely on the physical aspect of sex while ignoring its psychological aspect. The sex is shallow, emotionless, and unsatisfying for the woman.

Some guys don't mind being mediocre. Other guys want to improve and give women amazing sex (if you're reading this, then you're probably the latter). This leads us to the next important point...

The 3 Categories of Men

When it comes to sexual performance, there are 3 categories of men...

1) Men who don't give a shit about their performance in bed and never try to change anything.

These men are hopeless because they're not willing to try to improve. Most men fall into this category because they let their egos get in the way. It's too difficult for them to admit to themselves that they need help in the bedroom.

2) Men who are naturally great in bed.

These men know how to give women orgasm after orgasm with ease. But even these men can use a few tips now and then. There's always room to improve, even if you're already great in bed.

3) Men who want to improve, but usually don't go about it the right way.

These men recognize their need to improve in the bedroom but aren't quite sure how to go about it. They scour the web for the perfect sex position and how to hit the "G" spot.

If you're reading this, you may fall into the second category, but you probably fall into the third. And that's all good because you're finally going to learn how to improve the right way.

But what exactly is the "right way"?

Well, when the average guy tries to improve, he comes from a mindset that sex is purely a form of physical pleasure. He thinks that if he can just hit the right buttons and get into the right positons, she'll have mind-blowing orgasms and get addicted to him.

Here's the problem: women don't want a glorified

gynecologist going down on them and trying to pleasure them. They want to be fucked into submission by a dominant man.

And so, there are two important aspects involved. The physical and the psychological. In other words, you need to fuck her mind and her body if you want her to really feel pleasure.

How do you do that?

Well, that's exactly what you're about to learn.

The first step is to understand how women think about sex (because it's probably a lot different than the way you think about it).

Reference:

1. "New Survey: Most Women Are NOT Satisfied With Their Sex Lives." HealthyWomen. Accessed October 30, 2017. http://www.healthywomen.org/content/article/new -survey-most-women-are-not-satisfied-their-sex- lives.

How She Thinks About Sex (and How YOU Need To)

It's no secret that men and women view sex differently. To truly become great at sex, you'll have to understand how women view sex, too.

As a man, you can look at a girl and know within 3-5 seconds if you'd like to have sex with her.

As a woman, she can look at a guy and know within 3-5 seconds if sex is a *possibility*, but not if she'd definitely be willing to have sex with him. What's more, that 3-5 second "sex is a possibility" decision can shift quickly as well.

There's a lot more that goes into the decision for her than there is for you.

Why? Well, it's quite simple, really.

Men are programmed to be more conquest-oriented. We're programmed to want to fuck as many women as possible, spread our seed, and continue our bloodline.

There's less risk involved for us in a couple of big ways. Firstly (and perhaps most obviously), if we get a girl pregnant, we're not the ones who have to carry around the baby for 9 months. Hell, we can leave the next day, if we so choose, and be on to the next girl.

Secondly, it's a lot less risky in terms of how society will view us. It's no secret how society views promiscuity in men versus in women. The man looks awesome when he sleeps with a lot of women, while the girl is labeled as a slut.

Put simply: If a "perfect 10" girl slept with every guy who wanted to sleep with her, she'd no longer be a "perfect 10" in the eyes of society. She'd lose her mystique and value. In the process, she'd severely damage her ability to attract high quality men thanks to her reputation for sleeping with the whole city.

And so, the more promiscuous a girl is, the more difficult it'll be for her to find a quality guy to commit to her. And unlike us men who are more conquest-oriented, women are (usually) more commitment-oriented. They're programmed to want a high-quality guy who will stick around.

So it's quite a severe blow and can damage their chances of getting commitment from a high-quality guy.

Those are just a couple of the big risks from the woman's perspective (we'll talk about a few other risks in a minute).

But here's the thing: woman like sex just as much as (if not more than) men. So if you can show that you're a high-quality, authentic guy with a little charisma and dominance, many women will be open to sexual adventures with you.

You'll learn how to be that kind of guy in part II. But just being that kind of guy won't get women running to the bedroom with you.

That's because there's still one big problem:

Most men don't understand what women need before getting sexual with a guy. **If you don't give a woman what she needs before sex, then she's not going to want to have sex with you. She won't be ready.**

Now, of course, all women are different, and they have varying sexual preferences. Some women will be more willing to jump into bed with you quickly, while others will prefer to move more slowly. Despite these differences, though, there are 4 general things she needs from you before she'll have sex.

If you know what these things are, you'll be more aware of when a girl is (and isn't) ready to have sex. You'll also be able to adjust your approach to account for these things, so more women will be open to getting sexual with you.

The 4 Things She Needs from You Before Sex

1. She Needs to Feel Comfort and Trust With You.

Emotionally healthy women need to feel comfortable before sleeping with you. She must feel that you're not going to judge her or think she's a "slut," and also that you care about her well-being.

This comfort is also important to the actual quality of the sex. Women are turned on by the whole experience – not just the physical part of it. When she's comfortable with you, she'll allow herself to let go a little more and immerse herself in the sex.

So, how do you make women feel comfortable with you?

Refrain from stating judgmental opinions, especially about women.

Contentious and judgmental opinions are some of the worst conversation mistakes that turn women off. Instead, aim to be open and accepting in your conversations, and avoid the urge to make snap judgments.

And this is kind of obvious, but it's worth noting: you should refrain from talking about other women as "slutty" or generally talking badly about women for sleeping with other men. Because when you do this, she'll feel that you'll judge her if she chooses to have sex with you.

Actually care about her well-being.

A lot of guys aim to fuck women simply to add notches to their bed posts. Hell, that's how I used to be. Every time I bedded a new girl, the next number would tick off in my head. It took away from the experience and made me seem shallow and untrustworthy.

But you must avoid searching for this kind of validation (or extra notch) when you have sex with a woman. Instead, your motivation should lie in the desire to enjoy an amazing experience with her. She'll feel the difference, and it'll make her more comfortable around you.

Talk about emotional topics.

Emotional conversation topics lay the foundation for trust and a strong connection. These conversation topics should revolve around her, as the more she tells you about herself, the more she'll feel connected to you (and the more comfortable she'll be around you).

Here are some emotional conversation topics you can use:

- Her dreams

- Where she wants to travel

- Her career

- Her motivations

- What she loves to do

And once you hit on these, you can dive deeper by asking open-ended questions to continue the conversation.

These are questions like "What made you get into that?" and "What makes you want to travel there?"

Open-ended questions break a girl out of auto-pilot and require more than a simple yes or no response.

Overcome Her Objections.

Women will sometimes object to requests like going home with you and sleeping with you. The reason she objects usually has nothing to do with whether she actually wants to do the thing or not. In reality, it's more related to her social programming.

And that social programming usually tells her things like, "If I go home with this guy, my friends will judge me," or, "If I sleep with this guy on the first date, that must mean I'm slutty."

So if you can keep a cool head and overcome these objections (while of course recognizing that "no means no"), you can earn her trust and make her comfortable having sex with you.

Don't Be Desperate for Sex.

Women don't want to feel like you're desperate for sex. Yet the average guy signals exactly that.

When a girl says the typical, "You know we're not having sex tonight, right?," he gets reactive and offended. Even if he doesn't outright say so, the girl can tell that this has made him angry, and that he is indeed desperate for sex. This also signals that he probably doesn't have too much sex or an abundance of women in his life.

You should take the opposite approach and instead have a more relaxed attitude when it comes to sex. Sure, you'd like to have it, and it'd be a fun experience, but it's not the end of the world if you don't. When women see you have this relaxed attitude, they'll actually be a lot more comfortable having sex with you.

2. She Needs to Feel That It's Worth the Risk.

Women are very aware of the risks of sex – much more so than men. Here are some of the risks from their point of view:

- **The risk of getting pregnant.** I talked about this

before, and it's a big one. Obviously they're the ones who have to carry the baby if an accidental pregnancy happens.

- **The risk of STDs.** Most men are just carriers so they rarely experience physical effects related to STDs. On the other hand, Women are far more likely to be affected by STDs, as well as STD-induced diseases like different types of cancer.

- **The social risk that people will think she's a slut.** Whether it's right or wrong, our society tends to look down on women who have sex with a lot of different men.

- **The risk of an awkward sexual experience.** A lot of guys are terrible or mediocre at sex (hence the reason for this book), and she'd rather avoid those uncomfortable sexual experiences.

This risk awareness is also biological. This stems back to the hunter-gatherer days. If a woman got pregnant then, the man could leave her, and she'd be forced to fend for herself and her child in a tumultuous world.

Here's how to activate the feeling that it's worth the risk for her:

- **Make her comfortable around you**. (See the points from part I of this section.)

- **Always use protection.** This shows her that you're

not careless when it comes to sex and you understand the risks involved.

- Make a concerted effort to get to know her. Show genuine interest when she tells you about herself instead of just waiting for her to finish talking so you can talk more.

- Provide her with good emotions. The better she feels, the more likely she is to follow your lead as well as take things to the next level with you. So you should be leading her and managing her emotions throughout the interaction (you'll learn how to do this later).

3. She Needs to Feel Aroused.

She can trust you, feel comfortable with you, and feel like it's worth the risk, but if she doesn't feel aroused around you, then none of those things will matter.

That feeling of arousal breeds the desire for sex.

Throughout this book, you'll learn how to make women feel aroused. By developing your sexy vibe and applying the setup and foreplay fundamentals, you'll get women considering sex with you much more quickly than they do with other men.

For now, here's a snapshot of some things you can do to get her aroused:

- Escalate through "sexy talk" by speaking with intent and using sexual humor.

- Develop your sexy vibe so you become a naturally attractive man.

- Learn to read and act on the signs women give you.

4. She Needs You to Initiate It.

Women won't usually initiate sex. Again, there's too much social pressure. They want you to initiate it, as this removes the feeling of being a "slut" that society has ingrained in them. When you properly initiate it, she can rationalize it as, "I let go, and he led me to sex. I was just along for the ride."

Initiating things also shows masculinity and sexual confidence. Instead of waiting or hoping for sex to "just happen," you actively lead her along the journey in such a way that you both enjoy the experience.

Plus, leading her will turn her on and get her aroused. Throughout the process, you'll be infusing sexual undertones into the conversation and putting the idea of sex in her mind.

Here's what you can do to initiate things:

Make the Conversation More Sexual.

Throughout the conversation, you should introduce a

few sexual innuendos and jokes. The key is that you want to insinuate that sex is on the table without bluntly stating it. You also want to get her thinking of the possibility of sex with you.

A quick way to do this is to ask a question like, "What do you find sexy in a guy?"

Make the Move.

This is an obviously necessary part of initiating things. Usually girls won't make the first move, so the responsibility is on you. A good rule I like to go by is that when I feel like I want to make a move on a girl, I go for it. I don't force it because I think "it's the right time."

Remember: Every Woman Is Different

Like I said, all women are different, but these are the general things they need from you before they'll have sex.

Some women will need to feel a higher level of comfort, while others will just need to feel like you're a somewhat normal guy. As you work these things into your interactions more often, you'll get a better sense of which are more important for different types of women.

But you'll already be ahead of most guys who don't even take these things into account in the first place.

One more point to add: there's no specific "time limit" for these things. Some women will be ready for sex with you after an hour (or sometimes even less), while others will hold off until the second or third date (and maybe more, in some cases). But the better you are at achieving these 4 things, the quicker you'll be able to bed women.

Wrapping Up How She Thinks About Sex...

Most men play a guessing game when it comes to getting sexual with women. They don't have a great sense of when she's ready, and so they often make a move too soon or too late and miss their window. Or they miss these things completely and don't get her sexually interested at all.

If you follow along with this chapter and apply the knowledge in it, you can usually avoid these problems.

To recap, here are the 4 things she needs from you before sex:

1. She needs to feel comfort and trust with you.

2. She needs to feel that it's worth the risk.

3. She needs to feel aroused.

4. She needs you to initiate it.

Take these things into account on your dates and interactions with women. By doing so, more women will be open to getting sexual with you, and you'll both have a more enjoyable experience with each other.

A Note on the Female Orgasm

The female orgasm is an interesting thing. It has confused scientists for decades because they can't quite figure out its purpose.

It's not essential for successful reproduction, and yet, it still happens.

What's more, some women can have a seemingly infinite number of orgasms in one session of sex. Ten, twenty, or even more within an hour or less of sex. You'll be with some of these women, and if you perform well (which you will if you follow the advice in this book), then you'll see this phenomenon. It'll probably make you feel pretty good about yourself, too!

Some women, though, get very sensitive after one or two orgasms and need to take a break. Others struggle to even have one orgasm over the course of a whole session (even if it's good, and they enjoy it).

So, don't pat yourself on the back too much when you give a girl a lot of orgasms, and don't beat yourself up too much when you fail to give a girl one orgasm.

As you put the fundamentals you learn here into

practice, you'll learn more about each girl you sleep with. What she likes and dislikes, as well as her capacity for orgasms. And no matter how many orgasms she has within a given session (whether it be zero or twenty), the key is to focus on having an amazing overall experience.

Because sex isn't supposed to be just a means to achieve orgasm – it's a process meant to be enjoyed and fully experienced.

Part II: Developing Your Sexy Vibe

Sex Begins Long Before Penetration...

If you want to be great at sex, you must learn that sex is more than something you just "do."

It's a way of life. It's who you are.

You must become a sexual man and allow that sexuality to permeate your very being.

Because the truth is, sex begins long before penetration. Men who are great at sex understand this, while mediocre men are confused by it.

You see, sexual energy should seep into your every interaction with a girl... even from the moment you say "Hello."

The way you talk to women, the subtle jokes you make, the eye contact, the confidence... it is all colored by the hue of sexual energy. Sometimes just a hint; sometimes way, way more. It all depends on the situation.

I told you earlier that women can intuitively "sense" when a man is sexual and understands how to fuck a girl the right way. This is the reason they can sense it. And when they do sense it, they subconsciously separate you from 99% of other guys.

And when they separate you from 99% of other guys, they do things with you that they'd never do with 99% of other guys.

Threesomes, orgies, sex in club bathrooms, begging for you to come all over their face...

That's just the beginning.

You will see a different world of women that most men will only ever dream about. It's a world I've become familiar with over the past few years – a world where beautiful women eye me down before I even say a word, and a world where any sexual adventure is on the table.

Yes, you will become familiar with this world, too.

But that's ONLY if you can develop your sexy vibe.

And that's what Part II of this book is all about. You will learn how to become a sexual man who attracts and has sex with the women he wants. A man who takes initiative and doesn't hold back. A man who turns women on with a simple "hello" and a knowing grin.

So, read carefully, and don't be so quick to skip straight to the sex fundamentals. Because if you haven't mastered the fundamentals here, everything else will be all for naught.

The 4 Fundamentals of a Sexy Vibe

A coaching client of mine recently complained that women don't see him in a very "sexual" way.

They see him either as a friend or as the *provider* type that could make a good potential boyfriend *in the future*, but not as the *fun, sexy guy* they'd like to have an adventure with right now.

And so having casual sex has been somewhat of a challenge for him.

You may be familiar with this problem. It's common among many men.

If you don't have a sexy vibe, women don't usually see you in a sexual way. And so, it's a lot harder to have casual sex (if that's what you're after). Plus, it feels a little awkward when you make a move too quickly...

But if you can develop a sexy vibe around women, that will change.

You'll notice that women look at you in a different way, are more open to spontaneous adventures with you (like casual sex), and are instantly sexually attracted to you.

As I mentioned before, women will do things with you that they wouldn't dare try with "unsexy men," like have sex in the bathroom and go home with you the first night. Better yet, it will all feel natural (compared to the awkwardness of an average guy who tries to get sexual quickly).

How do you cultivate a sexy vibe around women? There are four fundamentals to this:

1. The surface level (what she can see). These are things you can physically do right now to cultivate a sexy vibe around women.

2. Your physical characteristics (how you appear). These are the components of your physical appearance, like your style and physique.

3. Under the hood (your personality characteristics). These are things you must develop and internalize over time.

4. The sexual mindsets. These are the mindsets that you must develop to become a sexual man.

You can do the surface level stuff now and sort of "fake it till you make it" until you fully develop the "under the hood" and mindset stuff. And the physical characteristics are not only a constant endeavor of improvement but also an enjoyable one.

The positive reinforcement you gain from the surface level stuff will make it easier to develop the rest.

Keep this in mind as we dive into these four fundamentals.

(And try not to get overwhelmed by all the pieces of a "sexy vibe." You can focus on one fundamental at a time. Once you master one, you'll internalize it, and you can move on to the next, until it becomes a part of who you are, and you don't even have to think about it.)

Fundamental #1: The "Surface Level" of Your Sexy Vibe

These are the physical steps you can take right now to have a sexy vibe.

The more you focus on them, the more positive reference experiences you will gain, and the easier it will be to develop the right mindsets and characteristics.

Focus on one at a time, and notice how each one changes the way you feel as well as the way women react to you.

Talk Slower

Picture the confident "bad boy" type of guy you see in movies, like James Bond. He's undoubtedly a character who has a sexy vibe around women.

Now ask yourself: how does he talk?

Does he speed through his sentences, hoping to get his words out before people get bored and stop listening?

No, right? He usually delivers his words slowly, and in

doing so, he captivates people. They hang on his words.

When you slow down your speech, you convey power and confidence. Plus, what you say seems more important.

So, talk slower than you think you should be talking, and then talk even slower. Experiment with it a bit and notice how people's reactions change.

It's the difference between a rushed, "HeyHow'sItGoing?!?!" and a calm and controlled, "Hey… How's it going?"

Move Slower

Powerful and sexy men also move slower.

Where an insecure man might walk fast and slouch with his head down, a sexy man will walk slowly down the street with his back straight, smiling at the women who pass by.

When you slow your movements down, you'll come off as more confident and sexually appealing.

This is especially important in a bar/club setting. Simply walking slowly and smiling will make women notice you, and they'll start giving you approach invitations.

(Approach invitations are a woman's way of letting

you know she wants you to approach her. This allows her to give you a sign that she likes you, without taking the social risk of literally approaching you and getting rejected, which is a bigger perceived social risk for women than it is for men.)

And when you approach them, the interaction will instantly have a sexual undertone.

Pause at the Right Time

Us guys tend to talk more and more when we get nervous. We're afraid that if we let the conversation die down, she'll get up and leave. So we go on and on, hoping to find a topic that interests the girl and strike up a good conversation.

Here's the problem: the point is not to get her interested in your choice of *topics*; it's to get her interested in *you*.

A well-timed pause builds sexual tension, allows her to invest in the interaction and talk about herself, and puts you in control of the pace of the conversation.

It also signals that you're confident and comfortable around women. Perhaps even better, it signals that you're in control – a trait that women love.

Here's when to pause:

- When you're considering the best way to say something.

- After she asks you a question.

- After asking intriguing questions.

- After you make a statement.

Hold Eye Contact

Eye contact is powerful — the brain sends out relationship-building chemicals like oxytocin when you make eye contact with somebody.

But you need to be able to make eye contact without being creepy.

When you're talking to women, focus on holding it for the majority of the time. Look at her right eye, so your eyes don't shift back and forth.

When you make eye contact, from the other side of the bar/club or even just in general, hold it until she looks away. Then, once you've made eye contact, walk towards her and approach her.

Good eye contact is something you must learn — so the more you practice, the better.

The Sexy Smile

Smiling is crucial, especially because of the

phenomenon of mirror neurons. Basically, these are brain cells that cause us to feel the same emotion as we see others feeling.

But you have to get your smile right.

Don't be like Urkel from *Family Matters*. Instead, aim for the type of smile that Ryan Gosling constantly uses in the movie *Crazy, Stupid, Love*.

Here are the characteristics of a "sexy" smile:

- Show very little of your teeth (or just keep your mouth shut).

- Smile with one side of your mouth more than the other.

- It's almost a "half smile" or slight grin, whereas the friendly guy's smile is very broad.

This is something you want to get down pat because many women will judge you based on your smile. If you're tired of being stuck in the friendzone, nail this one down.

Tone of Voice

Here's another tendency of nervous men: They talk with a higher-pitched voice. This is an instant turn-off for women and will get you labeled as 'just a friend'.

The problem is, when you're nervous, you tend to

speak from your throat.

Instead, practice speaking from your belly and projecting your voice.

To do this, focus on maintaining a deep breathing pattern. Breathe in through your nose and deep into your belly. You should feel your stomach rise and fall with each breath.

Practice this in private – that way, it feels more natural when you're with a girl.

We tend to speak from the same place we breathe from. If you breathe from your throat, you'll probably have a weak, high-pitched voice. But if you speak from your belly, your voice will likely be deeper and more masculine, which is essential for a good first impression.

Here's a quick recap of the "surface level" of your sexy vibe:

- Talk slower so you appear more confident and women hang on your words.

- Move slower to come across as more sexually appealing and controlled.

- Pause at the right time to build tension.

- Master the sexy smile instead of cheesing like Urkel.

- Deepen your tone of voice by speaking from your belly.

Now, let's move on to fundamental #2!

Fundamental #2: The Physical Level of Your Sexy Vibe

It is possible to have a sexy vibe around women without developing your physical characteristics. I have many friends who aren't traditionally "good-looking" who have plenty of success with women.

That being said, if you can improve your physical characteristics in the right way, your dating and sex life will become a lot easier. You'll get more "looks" from beautiful women, and some women will get turned on just by looking at you and touching your body.

For example, it's a lot easier to come off as a dominant and sexy man when you're a muscular guy than when you're a scrawny one. I used to be a scrawny guy, and I can attest to the difference.

And so, here are a few things you can do to improve your physical characteristics.

Work on Your Physique

When you're in shape, you'll look better, feel better, and have more energy to fuck a girl for as long as you want to.

I'm no fitness expert, so I won't dive deep into advice on this aspect. But I will say that simply lifting weights 2-3 times a week, doing some cardio (I prefer to do this in the form of pickup basketball), and eating a bit healthier can make a huge difference. There are plenty of resources online to show you how to do all 3 of these things.

In the span of a few years, I've gone from skinny to very muscular. I kid you not: I regularly catch women sneaking glimpses at my biceps while I'm talking to them, and I see the turned-on looks in their eyes when they hold onto my body and feel my abs.

And it's not like I'm some hulking dude either. I have a normal physique that errs on the side of muscular. And even that has made a huge difference.

So if you've been holding off on improving your physique, now is the time to get started.

Develop Your Style

I see dudes everywhere with pitifully bad style.

Here's the thing: A woman will judge you based on your style, even if she doesn't realize it. So if you look like a scrub, don't expect to attract sexy women on a consistent basis.

Again, I'm not a style expert here – but you don't need to be a style expert either.

Simply wear clothes that fit well!

My wardrobe consists of 5 V-neck shirts from Express, a few slim fit button-down shirts, some Lululemon shorts, and a couple of pairs of jeans from Mott & Bow (no affiliation – I just fucking love jeans from Mott & Bow. They're relatively cheap at around $100 and are super stretchy, comfortable, and stylish).

I also have one watch from Movement Watches, another brand I recommend because they have an awesome selection of watches, all at around $100 (but they look a lot more expensive).

Get a Good Haircut

Along with bad clothing styles, I see a lot of guys with terrible haircuts.

I speak from experience here... I had a buzz cut until I was 21 years old. Now, I grow my hair out more on top and cut it short on the sides, then gel it to one side. It's a more refined and unique look, and women like it a lot more.

I recommend checking out a quality salon in your area and asking for the booklet with all the pictures of haircuts. Talk to the stylist about what type of cut they think would suit you best, and experiment with it.

It took me a few tries to find my ideal hairstyle, but it was well worth it.

Building on this point, make sure to have your facial hair looking good, too. If you're a beard guy, grow a beard, but keep it trimmed and well-maintained.

Again, experiment with different types of facial hair and figure out what kind of style you like best. Be sure to ask the women in your life which style looks the best, too, so you can get an objective perspective from a woman.

Here's a quick recap of the "physical level" of your sexy vibe:

- Work on your physique so you look better and have more sexual stamina.

- Develop your style and wear clothes that fit well.

- Get a good haircut to be more physically appealing, and keep your facial hair well-groomed.

Fundamental #3: The Deeper Aspect of Your Sexy Vibe

These are characteristics you will develop over time. These are the things that women truly want in a man.

When you combine these with the surface level and physical stuff, you'll be much closer to having a sexy vibe that puts you ahead of 99% of men – and it will make women excited to have sex with you.

Here are the characteristics that women fawn over…

Charisma

This trait can make you magnetic to people (and especially to women). Charisma is essentially the magical *"something"* that you can't seem to put your finger on, but it draws people in and gets them interested. It's charming and intriguing.

And most importantly, it's incredibly sexy to women.

There are four important factors to developing

charisma:

1. Certainty. Charismatic people are sure of themselves and their actions. So you need to believe in what you're saying and speak with certainty. This is especially important if you want women to follow your lead.

2. Presence. Charismatic people are fully in the moment. They're not glancing at their phones every few minutes, ignoring your words to further prove a point, or faking their interest. They genuinely care about what you're saying and approach the interaction with an open sense of curiosity.

3. Warmth. Charismatic people are warm - they immediately bring people into their world and treat them well. When you approach a girl, come from the mindset that you've known her for a long time – that you're comfortable with her. This "instant friendship" type of vibe will amplify her trust in you and make the conversation go smoothly.

4. Low Filter. Charismatic people don't let their actions be affected by what others will think of them. Many guys hold back from cracking a joke, or making a sexual innuendo, for fear of what the girl will think of them. Instead, be more unfiltered with your words and actions. Understand that no matter the outcome, life will go on.

Authentic Sense of Humor

Women want a man who has a good attitude, can laugh at himself and the world around him, and doesn't get easily offended.

You can be that man by developing an authentic sense of humor.

This doesn't mean you're great at telling jokes, or that you're a stand-up comedian. It means that you can appreciate jokes, find humor in different situations, and be self-amused.

Here are some ways you can develop a good sense of humor:

- Go to stand-up comedy shows and watch comedians on YouTube/Netflix.

- Watch comedy movies and TV series with different kinds of humor, like Adam Sandler movies, *The Office*, and *Rick and Morty*.

- Observe people in your own life with good senses of humor and learn from them.

- Aim to approach life with a generally good-natured attitude. Catch yourself if you can feel you're getting offended a bit too easily, find the light in dark situations, and avoid taking yourself so seriously all the time.

- Learn how to tease women the right way (you can check out my book, Conversation Casanova where I cover that in-depth).

Independence

Women want a man who doesn't need anybody in order to achieve happiness or success.

Because if a man can't survive on his own and fails to be independent, then he cannot lead his woman. He is weak, and his life will be a constant stream of failures and disappointments. High quality women know this.

So, how can you be more independent?

- **Become self-reliant.** Take on problems in your life with an open sense of curiosity. You may not know the solution or have much experience dealing with the particular problem at hand, but don't let that stop you. Educate yourself on the problem, think through a set of solutions, and experiment.

- **Be accountable for your life.** Most people go through life with a "victim mentality." They blame other people and things for their own lack of success instead of figuring out what they can do to change things. Never allow yourself to fall into a victim mentality. Remember that the only person that can save you is yourself. The only person that determines your success is you. Armed with this knowledge, set out to create a life that excites you at your very core.

- **Don't let your emotions control you.** Take a balanced view of the world and the problems you face. Step back and aim to see things objectively instead of letting your emotions swing you from one direction to the other, as so many weak-minded people tend to do. To be a sexy man, you must have control over your own state of mind.

Purpose

The way you fuck the world is the way you fuck your girl.

This is why women crave men with purpose. They want a man who delivers his gifts onto the world, know what he wants, and goes for it.

But most men don't live a life of purpose. They are easily swayed by the winds of each day, wilt at the smallest sense that something is wrong, fall into quarter-life and mid-life crises, and never seize control of the gift they've been given – the gift of life.

These men are quick to make women their top priority and rely on them for their happiness. And so, they are also the quickest to get bitter when they feel like women have treated them wrong.

But women want a man who has greater aspirations than simply being with them.

The question is, do you know your purpose? Do you wake up every day with a sense of excitement to conquer the next task at hand? Or has life become a saga of let-downs and what ifs?

If you're not sure if you're living a life of purpose, ask yourself these 4 questions:

- *"What lights my fire and makes me come alive?"*

- *"What is a problem in the world that I can help solve?"*

- *"By what metrics will I measure my life?"*

- *"What are my greatest values?"*

Having a purpose will help you ravish women in the bedroom, and it will turn them on like you won't believe. They will feel the difference.

But living by your purpose will benefit your life in many more ways than just that, as you will see along your own journey.

Remember: The way you fuck the world is the way you fuck your girl.

Here's a quick recap of the deeper aspect of your sexy vibe:

- Develop your charisma so that you come off as more interesting, intriguing, and sexy.

- Develop an authentic sense of humor so that you look at life positively and have a good attitude.

- Become more independent and stop relying on other people for your own happiness.

- Live a purposeful life so that you have greater aspirations than simply being with a woman.

Fundamental #4: The Sexual Mindsets

Your sexual mindsets are the final aspect of your sexy vibe. They separate you from the shallow men who manipulate women and use them for sex.

Instead, they allow you to truly enjoy your experience with women and provide a much better experience for every girl you sleep with.

Because make no mistake: We're not trying to "take" something from women here. We're trying to give them an amazing sexual experience.

And so, these mindsets will help you keep a level head as you continue to improve in the bedroom and also help you to treat women well along the way (so they feel good about having been with you).

A bonus of these mindsets is that they'll actually lead to having a lot more sex with women, too.

"I Can Enjoy a Woman's Presence Without the Need for Sex."

"Are you going to be angry with me if we don't have sex?"

I've gotten this question from several women while

taking them home for the first time.

They don't ask this question because of anything I've done or said. They ask it because they know what the expectations could be if they come home with me (i.e. having sex), and they've had other guys get frustrated and angry when they've thwarted their attempts at sex in this situation.

So they're afraid that if they come back and don't have sex with me, I'll get mad like so many other guys have.

They're usually surprised to discover that I have the opposite reaction. Sure, I like to have sex with beautiful women. But if it doesn't happen on one particular night, I'm perfectly fine with it.

I can enjoy her presence without the need for sex.

This acceptance puts the girl at ease because she doesn't feel the pressure of needing to have sex. And usually, this ends up leading her to have sex with me in the end anyway, and she's happy she did.

So, how do you develop this mindset?

There are 2 ways:

1) See the woman as an end in herself and not simply a means to get sex. Embrace and enjoy her feminine presence, and immerse yourself in the experience of being around her. That can be refreshing and exhilarating in itself.

2) Develop an attitude of abundance toward women. When you know you can meet and attract beautiful women with relative ease, you know it's not the end of the world if you don't have sex with one beautiful girl on a particular night. Of course, developing an attitude of abundance toward women is easier said than done, but I've already created plenty of resources to help you do that (and a whole host of articles on my website, **www.postgradcasanova.com)**.

And here's an example of what you can say to a girl to demonstrate this mindset:

If she says something like, "You know we're not having sex tonight, right?" or, "We can go back to your place, but no sex," then you can say, "That's cool, I don't have any expectations." This puts her at ease and makes her feel like she's not opting into some unspoken contract to have sex with you if she goes back to your place.

"I Won't Always Perform at My Best Sexually, and That's Okay."

No matter how great you get at sex, and no matter how much you master the fundamentals in this book, there will be times when you come up short in the bedroom.

Perhaps you have trouble getting it up, finish in a minute or two, or simply don't put on your best performance.

That's okay, it happens. Even if you can perform well most of the time, you'll occasionally slip up. Nobody is perfect.

And so, a mindset like this is key. It allows you to accept the fact you won't always have great sex every time, which takes pressure off of you. You'll no longer feel like it's the end of the world if you finish in two minutes. And if something like this does happen, you'll react calmly, and the girl won't feel like it's a big deal either.

The result? You're in your own head less, and you can focus on enjoying great sex with the girl.

One of the best ways to develop this mindset is to not take yourself too seriously.

If you take yourself too seriously, one slip-up can cause you to question yourself and your ability, and you'll end up in a sexual rut. It'll go from a one-time mishap to a cycle of average or below-average sex. You'll be in your head and question yourself.

Instead, recognize that things like this are a part of life, and that it's okay. You don't need to beat yourself up for one subpar performance.

Also recognize that as you improve in the bedroom,

you might have some awkward "learning" moments along the way, but it's all part of the experience. And each of those learning moments will help you improve in the long run, and hey, they may even make for some funny stories to look back on.

"I Can Give Women an Amazing Sexual Experience."

Many men have low or average sexual confidence. They're not certain about their ability to pleasure a woman in the bedroom, nor their ability to give her an unforgettable experience.

If you're uncertain about your sexual ability, girls will pick up on it. She'll notice how you hesitate to lead her, lack dominance, and fail to infuse sexuality into the conversation. You'll also tend to subconsciously sabotage yourself in your interactions so that you prevent sex from even happening.

The mindset of, "I can give women an amazing sexual experience," is the opposite of that uncertainty. It allows you to treat her like a sexual man and lead her through the stages of an interaction (and eventually into the bedroom) with confidence.

Not only will it make you better at sex, but it'll also help you to have more sex in general.

The best way to develop this mindset is to actively try to learn and improve your sexual ability.

If you're not naturally great at sex (and most guys aren't), then you have two choices. You can 1) hope that you randomly improve as you get older, or 2) actively try to learn and improve so that it's no longer a matter of chance.

You should take the active route – and if you're listening to this now, then you're already on the right path. Apply the fundamentals you learn, try new techniques, and have authentic conversations with the women you sleep with

Approach sex with an open mind and check your ego. Be willing to take feedback from women and ask questions to more experienced guys.

Here's a quick recap of the sexual mindsets:

- "I can enjoy a woman's presence without the need for sex."

 - "I won't always perform at my best, and that's okay."

- "I can give women an amazing sexual experience."

Part III: The "Setup" Fundamentals (Turn Her On and Get Her Ready)

Without the "Setup," You Can't Close...

You might be wondering, "What is the 'setup,' and why is it important for great sex?"

The setup is all the things that lead up to the actual sexual experience with a woman.

The way you lead her, talk to her, kiss her, turn her on, and even the way you set up your bedroom...

These things set the stage for great sex. Without them, you likely won't even get to the "sex part" with a girl, and if you do, it won't be nearly as good as it could've been.

And yes, this holds true whether you're in a relationship with a girl or just having sex with her for the first time.

Remember: You need to fuck her mind AND her body. These fundamentals will help you turn her on both mentally and physically so she's ready and excited to take things further with you.

Let's get right into these setup fundamentals...

Fundamental #5: Escalate Through "Sexy Talk"

Your words are powerful – especially when talking to a woman.

They can make the difference between giving a conversation a platonic vibe or a subtly sexual one.

And that difference alone can get a woman thinking about sex with you – or at least not ruling the idea out.

Your words can also turn her on so that she's ready for sex when the time comes.

So, how do you escalate through sexy talk in your conversations?

Here are four great ways to do it...

Sexual Humor

Sexual humor is great for adding a sexual undertone to the conversation. The point is to plant the idea of you and her doing things together, or at the very least, get her thinking of sex around you.

An easy way to get started is to reinterpret

something she said, or something from the conversation in general, and make it sexual.

Note: Before using sexual humor, you should have built at least a little rapport with her. Otherwise, it can come off as a little creepy. The more you try to use sexual humor, the better you'll get at this.

The delivery is key here — you should have a sly, ironic sort of smile. You want her to know that you're joking, but also that you're comfortable with the subject of sex.

And I assure you, with a little creativity, you can turn almost any topic into sexual humor.

Here are a few examples of sexual humor in action...

Let's say you're talking about dancing (you can push the conversation in this direction by asking if she knows salsa or bachata). You could joke around about how you have a lot of rhythm, and how rhythm is important for a lot of things, not just dancing (obviously hinting that it's important for sex, too, without saying it outright).

Let's say she's a little bit older than you. You can tell her that you like older women because they know what they want, and they have a lot of experience in some important areas. Here, you're hinting that she knows what she wants in the bedroom, and also that she's good in bed.

Notice how each of these is subtle. You don't come right out and say, "I have good rhythm, so I can fuck you well." Instead, you imply that rhythm is important for sex without actually saying it. The subtlety is key – it's more socially savvy, keeps her on her toes, and is more intriguing.

Self-amusement is also key here – you want to have fun with it. If you think it's funny and a little sexual, be unfiltered and go for it.

Speak with Intent

You usually approach a girl because you're attracted to her. There's something about her that you find sexy. But throughout your whole life, you've been programmed to cover up your sexual desires. You've basically been told to hide the fact that you have a dick, thanks to all the crappy advice and political correctness in the media.

But you do have a dick, so you should act like you fucking have one. The girl should have no doubt that she's speaking to a sexual man who goes for what he wants.

Your intent should come through in all the words you say. Even if you ask, *"Do you know where the nearest Starbucks is?,"* you want to sub-communicate something like, *"I think you're sexy, and I want to know more."*

On the surface, here's what it looks like to communicate with intent:

- Hold strong eye contact

- Speak from your stomach with a deeper tone of voice

- Talk slower

- Smile

Below the surface, you're thinking:

- I might want to have sex with this girl, and I'm okay if she picks up on this vibe

- She's attracted to me

This takes some work, but once you can start communicating with intent, your conversations with women will transform.

Look at Her Lips

Infusing a sexual undertone isn't just about the words you say. It's also about your behavior within the interaction.

One thing you can do to add a little sexiness to the vibe is to look at her lips.

While she's talking to you, glance slowly down at her lips for a second, and then back up to her eyes. Do this a few times throughout the conversation. Don't be blatant about it, but do it just subtly enough for her to notice.

No matter what you're talking about, this simple lip glance can her thinking of intimacy with you. It amplifies the vibe, and if she returns the glance and looks at your lips, then you know it's probably ON. I've been doing this more and more on dates recently and it really does make a difference.

Connect on a Deeper Level

This one isn't as inherently "sexual" as the previous three, but it is important in terms of the verbal build up. Think back to the chapter about how she thinks about sex. Remember how women need to trust you, feel comfortable with you, and feel that it's worth the risk before having sex with you…

Well, a big way to do all three of those things is to connect with her on a deeper level.

That means getting past the platonic "niceties" of small talk and drilling down to the stuff that really matters…

The way she feels about things, what she wants to do with her life, what she finds sexy in a guy, what she's passionate about, etc.

The more you discover about topics like these, the more connected she'll feel to you. Just make sure to listen closely and relate back with experiences and things from your own life.

For example, after she tells you what she finds sexy in a guy, you should tell her what you find sexy in a girl. After she tells you what she's passionate about, perhaps you can tell a story of your experience with one of those passions.

Whatever the case, the more you do this, the deeper the connection will be, and the better the sex will be when you get to that point.

Here's a quick recap of escalating through "sexy talk":

- Use sexual humor — but remember to be subtle and throw in the occasional innuendo.

- Speak with intent to convey your sexual vibe and turn her on.

- Look at her lips to get her thinking about sex.

- Connect on a deeper level to earn her trust and make the sex better later on.

Fundamental #6: Recognize When She's Horny (and Wants You to Make a Move)

You're out with a girl, and the two of you are really hitting it off.

Maybe you just met her at the bar, or the two of you are having first date drinks. Whatever the case, you like her, she appears to like you, and you'd like to take her home (or at least make a move).

But if you're like most guys, this is the point where you screw things up. It's mostly due to the fact that you're not 100% sure if she wants you to make a move, and you don't know what signs to look for.

She very well may be ready, but if you wait too long, the window will close, and you'll lose your opportunity.

But since you don't want to screw it up, you sit back and play it safe. You think to yourself:

"Now isn't the right time. If I try to make a move now, it might turn her off and screw up the whole interaction. Instead, I'm going to wait until it's really obvious and then make my move."

*(**Note:** There is no "right time" to make a move. As you get more experience with women, you'll begin to recognize that the best time to make a move is usually when you feel the urge to make a move. Until you get enough experience, though, it's a huge help to know the right signs to look for.)*

What usually happens next is a mix of the following:

- Stalling and having platonic conversations.

- One or both of you will get overly tired and want to go home (alone).

- Another guy will spot the window, swoop in, and take her home.

Overall, the interaction will stall, and you'll probably lose your chance.

The problem is, most women won't straight up tell you, "Let's go back to your place" or "Make the move!" There's too much social pressure for her. So you need to know how to spot her signals that she wants you to make a move.

If you can learn these signals, you'll stop missing opportunities with girls who want to go home and sleep with you and start making your move before the "hook up" window closes.

So here are some big signs that she's horny and possibly wants to go home with you right now...

*(**Note:** Some girls may be ready to leave with you within the first 5 minutes of talking, while others won't be ready for 2+ hours. Don't get caught up on the timing – instead, pay attention to the signals.)*

She's Receptive to Your Touch and Touches You Back

Physical touch is one of the most important parts of connecting with a woman. If you know how to touch her during conversation, you can turn her on and get her thinking of sex.

Here are some tips for touching her the right way:

- The best places to touch her are her elbow, upper arm, and the small of her back.

- Touch her early in the conversation (you can do something simple like a handshake introduction).

- Touch her at high points (like when the two of you are laughing, or she's agreeing with you).

*(For more on how to touch her during conversation, check out the chapter called "Flirting Without Your Words" in my book **Conversation Casanova.**)*

Now, if she's receptive to your touch (i.e. she welcomes it and doesn't tense up), then she probably feels comfortable with you. If she starts touching you back, then she's probably sexually attracted to you.

It's a clear sign that she's open to the idea of you making a move – and maybe even going home with you.

(Note: You can test her receptiveness by holding her hand when walking between venues. Does she hold on and even squeeze your hand back?)

She Gets in Your Personal Space (and Is Comfortable with You in Hers)

If you're in her "bubble," and she's okay with it, that's a sign that she either doesn't have many personal boundaries, or she's really interested in you (let's assume the latter).

The same goes for if she gets in your personal bubble. She probably won't do it unless she's interested in you.

When you get in each other's personal bubbles, the sexual tension skyrockets. However, if you don't make your move, it will eventually dissipate. So be aware of this one and be prepared to invite her home.

She Talks Less and Gives Shorter Answers

You've been hanging with her a bit, and you can feel the connection. At this point, it's clear that she's at least somewhat into you.

Suddenly, you notice she talks less and gives shorter answers. You can tell it's not for lack of interest, but more out of a sense of anticipation. Like she wants you to move things along without blatantly saying so.

So, that's exactly what you need to do. The window is open, and you need to make your move and invite her home. The longer you wait to do so, the quicker the window will close.

The Two of You Are Alone in Private

This one seems obvious - but when you're in private with a girl and she's not giving you any of the other signals we've talked about, it can still seem like the wrong time to make a move.

But in this case, the setting itself is the biggest signal of all. Odds are, she won't allow the two of you to be alone in private unless she's comfortable with the idea of hooking up with you.

She might not be down to have sex just yet, but at the very least, she's aware that that is a possibility when she goes home with you.

So if the two of you are alone in private, keep this in mind. Even if it seems like it's "not the right time," you might as well go for it. She wouldn't be there if she wasn't at least somewhat interested in you.

(As a general rule, you should make a move within ten to twenty minutes of being in private with a girl.)

She Holds Lingering Eye Contact

She doesn't just hold eye contact while she's talking to you... she also lets her eye contact linger during pauses.

Perhaps she even lowers her eyelids a little bit and gives you "bedroom eyes."

This is one of the clearest signs that she wants you to make a move. Get ready to invite her back to your place.

She Asks About Your Living Situation

"Do you have roommates?"

Whenever she asks a question like this, a bell should go off in your head.

Even if she doesn't realize it, this is a sign that she's subconsciously thinking about going home with you. The question is an attempt to get a feel for your living situation and see if she'd have to deal with anybody else if she goes with you.

She Complies With Your Requests

This is another tell-tale sign that she's horny, willing to follow your lead, and open to the idea of going home with you.

When she complies with your requests, it shows that she's interested in you and trusts that you can lead her to a fun and satisfying experience. Of course, there are different levels of compliance, and you can start slow when you test these out.

For example, if you meet her on the dance floor, you can take her hand and say, "Let's go hang by the bar." Then, once you've hung out for a little bit, you can say, "Let's go outside for a minute and get some fresh air."

And finally, you can say, "I live close by, let's go back to my place for a drink."

The more she complies and the bigger the requests that she complies to, the hornier she is and the more open she is for sex with you.

She Checks You Out

You notice her eyes drift a bit to your body. Maybe she sneaks a glance at your biceps, or takes a quick look at your lips. Whatever the case, she's subtly (or, perhaps, not so subtly) checking you out.

Women are good at sneaking these glances, so it takes some awareness to notice them. But if you do catch her, then you've got a clear sign that she's horny.

Now, you might be wondering, "Once it's time to make the move, how do I do it the right way?"

For that, you need to become a great kisser. And that's what we'll talk about next.

But first, here's a quick recap of the signs that she's horny (and wants you to make a move):

- She's receptive to your touch and touches you back.

- She gets in your personal space (and is comfortable with you in hers).

- She talks less and gives shorter answers.

- The two of you are alone in private.

- She holds lingering eye contact or checks you out.

- She complies with your requests.

Fundamental #7: Turn Her On from the First Kiss (and Get Her Thinking About Sex)

We sat in the movie theater holding hands.

I could feel her glancing at me from the corner of my eye. It was obvious that she wanted me to move in for the kiss (and also obvious that she had more experience with this stuff than me, even though she was a year younger).

I ignored her glances for as long as possible because I had no idea how to kiss a girl. I felt like if I kissed her, I'd be exposed. How could a 10th grader still not know how to kiss a girl?!

Some friends had told me that you just need to "stick your tongue in her mouth and move it clockwise." That's about the only knowledge I had to go off of.

I couldn't ignore her sideways glances for any longer without feeling like a wuss. So I checked my ego and went in for the kiss.

I went for it just like my friends had told me to. I stuck my tongue right in there and turned it clockwise and counterclockwise, attacking her mouth like a cyclone. "This is easy!" I thought. "I'm really getting the hang of this!"

I thought for sure I was doing a great job, and she seemed to like it, too.

***

A few hours later, I sat down at home, excited. I'd finally kissed a girl and done it well.

Then a message popped up on my computer. It was her…

"I just want to tell you… You are one HELL of a bad kisser."

My heart dropped. Apparently, I still didn't have the slightest idea of how to kiss a girl.

That's when I began to realize just how important kissing really is…

***

The way you kiss tells a woman a lot about the way you have sex.

If you're careless and not in the moment, she'll assume you're the same way in bed.

But if you give her a passionate, dominant kiss, you'll get her wet with anticipation.

In this chapter, I'll talk about how to become a great kisser so you can turn her on from the first kiss...

How to Go in for the First Kiss

First, you should understand that different environments call for different types of kisses. For example, your kiss in a nightclub should be different than your kiss in the bedroom.

More specifically, you should kiss a girl differently in situations where sex is immediately possible (like when you're in a bedroom or a private place) versus when it is not (like when you're at a bar or some other public place).

I'll talk first about how to kiss a girl in a public place. These will be the bulk of your first kisses with women.

When kissing a girl in a situation where sex is possible, you can start right off with the sexual kiss (which you'll learn about in a minute).

Here's how to go in for a normal first kiss...

- **Pause and look into her eyes.** Stop talking for a couple of seconds and look into her eyes. Lower your eyelids slightly and notice what you find sexy about her. This will make your eye contact more sexual.

- **Pull her in physically.** Hold her by the small of her back and gently pull her in towards you with one hand.

- **Start the kiss lightly, with low intensity.** Go in light – this will allow you to gradually build up to a deeper kiss.

- **Lightly nibble on her lip.** Gently nibble on her lower lip. Make sure to do it lightly; otherwise you might give her a fat lip, which is a bigtime mood killer.

- **Use a little bit of tongue.** Open your mouth slightly and use a little bit of tongue. Don't jam it in there like a cyclone (like I used to do). Instead, use it lightly and just kind of poke it in a little bit to give her a preview.

- **Be the first to pull away (after 5-10 seconds).** You don't need a full-on 5 minute long make-out session here. Maintain control and keep the sexual tension alive by being the first one to pull away.

The goal here is not just to enjoy the kiss but also to use it to build sexual tension. Where other men want to keep kissing her for minutes at a time and give all of the control and validation to the girl, you don't give in so easily. You maintain control by being the first one to pull back, and also by avoiding giving her your "full kiss." It's better to save that for the sexual kiss that we're going to talk about next.

The result? You keep her intrigued and wanting

more. Instead of defusing the sexual tension (which typically happens after one or two long make-out sessions because the girl is now 100% sure that you want to fuck her), you actually create more sexual tension. You tease her with a small kiss and get her thinking about the big passionate kiss that could be coming soon.

And that passionate kiss is what we'll talk about next...

Mastering the "Sexual" Kiss

After you tease her with "normal kisses" throughout the night, you can transition to a sexual kiss once sex is on the table (i.e. the two of you are back at your place or hers).

This kiss basically leads right into sex. It's intense, sexual, and has lots of intimate, physical contact. You're finally giving her the "full kiss" she's been craving all night.

Here's how to master the sexual kiss and turn her on...

- **Grab and hold her hair from the roots.** The majority of women love dominant men, and so they like it at least a little bit rough. When you hold her hair from the roots while kissing her, it shows that you're a dominant man and will often turn her on even more. Note that you don't need to hold your hand there the whole time – you can switch back and forth, first holding it for a few seconds and causing her to tilt her head, and then letting it go.

- **Tilt your head at a deeper angle.** With the normal kiss, you only need to tilt your head enough to not bump her nose straight on, because you're not going for a deep kiss. But the sexual kiss is more passionate and deep, and to get deeper, you'll need to tilt your head more than before.

- **Hold her more tightly.** Bring her in with a little more force than with the normal kiss. Then, hold her more tightly while kissing her. The increased physical contact will turn her on and make the kiss more passionate.

- **Open your mouth wider.** You only slightly opened your mouth and used a little bit of tongue with the normal kiss. But here, you'll open it a bit more widely (not all the way – you're not at the dentist's here) and use more tongue. This makes the kiss more intense and sexual. When you use your tongue, use it in a playful way with hers. You can lick her tongue, flick it with the tip of your own, and explore her mouth a little bit.

- **Suck on her tongue.** This is a technique I learned from one of my first college girlfriends. It works like this: when her tongue is in your mouth, close your lips on it and suck lightly. Do it for just a second or two – that's all you'll need. It adds some uniqueness and intensity to the kiss, and it shows her that you're savvy in this area.

- **Kiss her ears and neck**. Pull back occasionally and kiss her neck and ears. You can even give her a gentle bite as well – just try not to make a mark and give her a hickey (unless you want her to give you one in return). Kissing her neck and ears like this is a great way to turn her on and start transitioning into sex.

- **Pick her up and have her wrap her legs around you.** This is one of the best ways to transition from the sexual kiss into actually having sex. In the midst of the kiss, you pick her up, put her legs around you, and walk her to the bed.

Wrapping Up How to Turn Her On from the First Kiss...

Women will judge you by the quality of your kissing, so you need to get good at it. Otherwise, you'll turn women off with your kiss instead of getting them amped up for sex.

The first kiss will usually be in a public place. So here you'll want to use the kiss to build sexual tension and maintain control of the situation. Because if you go for the sexual kiss, you'll defuse the tension and give her too much validation, at which point sex will become unlikely.

The sexual kiss is the one you should save for when

sex is on the table (i.e. the two of you are in private). It amplifies the sexual tension, gets her extremely turned on, and can easily be transitioned into sex.

Fundamental #8: Transform Your Apartment into a Panty-Dropping Bachelor Pad

Preparation is the key to success in almost every area...

...and that's especially true when it comes to the dating and sexual realms.

And yet most guys completely ignore preparation. They don't bother to learn how to have better conversations with women, how to develop their sexy vibe, or how to make a great first impression.

So it's no surprise that they also don't bother to prepare their apartment in a way that gives them the best chance of sleeping with a girl (or, at the very least, not scaring her off).

While having a panty-dropping bachelor pad isn't the most important element of attracting women, it will make things a whole lot easier for you.

(By the way, by "panty-dropping," I mean it makes women want to drop their panties and sleep with you when they walk in.)

I'm speaking from experience here because I've been on both ends of the spectrum: shitty, uncomfortable apartment/bedroom, and panty-dropping bachelor pad. I promise you the latter is much better, and the former cock-blocked me more times than I can count.

In short, you should have this handled. It will make your game better and your life easier.

Before we get started, you should know the four necessary elements of a panty-dropping bachelor pad:

- Cleanliness

- Ambiance

- Comfort

- Preparedness

You'll learn about each of these elements in this chapter.

*(**Note:** You should make sure you have all this handled before you go on a date or out to a bar/club, because you never know when you'll be bringing a girl back to your place.)*

Now let's talk about exactly how you can transform your apartment into a panty-dropping bachelor pad...

Element #1: Cleanliness

When it comes to hygiene and cleanliness, women probably notice more than you. And odds are they won't be comfortable in a messy, disorganized apartment. For some women, this is even a big turn off. So let's talk about how to master the cleanliness element.

Make Your Bed

I don't like making my bed. It's annoying, and I don't really care if it's made or not. If I had it my way, I'd leave the sheets crumpled up, and I'd happily hop into bed just like that (sorry, mom).

But whenever I suspect I might have a lady friend over, I always make my bed – and you should, too.

Not only does it make your pad seem cleaner and feel more comfortable, it's also a lot more enticing to hop into bed.

Clean Your Room and Bathroom

When she excuses herself to go to your bathroom after walking in, she's usually not just... you know...

peeing.

She's also subconsciously (or consciously, for some women) taking note of the cleanliness. Is your toilet seat up? Are there shaving accessories and other things scattered across the counter?

Aim to make your bathroom as clean and as organized as possible because women will judge you for it whether they verbally tell you or not.

The same goes for your bedroom. You shouldn't have clothes strewn across the floor or shoes scattered around. Your mom was onto something when she told you to clean your room when you were a kid.

Wash Your Dishes

Occasionally you'll prepare drinks for your female guest. And for that, you'll need to be in the kitchen. If you have dirty plates and glasses stacked up, it's not a good sign.

Instead, make it a point to clean your dishes before women come over. Personally, I clean my dishes after each meal. It makes it easier to manage – and I don't have to stare down a big stack of dishes every night. I suggest you do the same.

Element #2: Comfort

A woman's level of comfort is a big factor in whether

or not she'll sleep with you. So the more comfortable your bachelor pad, the better you'll be able to seduce her.

Here's how you can make it more comfortable:

Get Comfortable Bedding

Your bed should be littered with comfortable pillows and a nicely designed, fluffy comforter. There are many types of mattresses out there, so that's up to you and what you sleep best on.

But the sheets add a high level of comfort to the bed – so make sure you have nice sheets and lots of pillows. A nice design doesn't hurt either (I'd advise against all white sheets because, well, you know…).

As a side note, you should also wash your bedsheets at least once a week – not once a month, like we've all probably been doing.

Have the Right Size Bed

At the absolute smallest, you should have a full-sized bed. Overall, the bigger, the better, and king size is the best.

Ideally, both of you will be able to lie down and stretch out on the bed.

What's more, a bigger bed allows for more positions… if you catch my drift.

I've stayed at Airbnbs across the world, and occasionally, I've been stuck with a twin bed. I can assure you it's the absolute worst for sex, and if the girl wants to sleep over, you're in for an uncomfortable night.

Element #3: Ambiance

Ambiance is absolutely crucial. I might even say it's the most important element to your bachelor pad, and it's especially important in the bedroom. The ambiance mainly consists of the lighting and music. Both of these things set the mood for the apartment and the bedroom.

Have a Music Speaker (with Bass If Possible)

You don't need a fully equipped sound system, but you do at least need a speaker. I travel a lot, so I have a small portable speaker from *JBL Go*. It fits in the palm of my hand, and it's plenty loud enough to play good music and set the mood.

If you're not constantly on the road, you may want to invest in a slightly better speaker system with some bass. This helps set the mood as well.

The reason for the speaker (and the music itself) is that 1) it blocks out outside noise (which can be distracting and a mood-killer), and 2) it disengages the logical mind and makes you and the girl more present.

Have a Good Playlist Ready

Your speaker system doesn't matter if you play shitty music.

I messed around for a long time trying to find a good hook up playlist. I use Spotify, and there are tons of playlists available. For a while, I used my own main playlist, but I have the occasional hilarious girly song in there, and it throws off the mood (don't worry, Alanis Morissette – you still my girl).

Earlier this year, I came across a much better playlist. It's called "Chill Vibes." It has tons of chill, laid back songs that are perfect for setting the mood and hooking up. Just search "Chill Vibes" on Spotify playlists, and you can check it out. I suggest queuing this up right after you get home with a girl.

But if you're planning to have some intense rough sex, then something a little less chill, like hardcore rap or metal, can also be good. It's ok to switch things up and go with different playlists for different moods and different styles of sex.

Warm Lighting

When you walk into your bedroom, it shouldn't feel like you just stepped foot into Forever 21.

Warm lighting is the way to go. Most overhead lighting is too bright, so I suggest getting a lamp with some warmer light. You can even get scented candles and incense, which are both a great way to set the mood.

Another alternative, though, is a laser or an LED disco ball.

Yes, you heard me right, and yes, I use this.

You can set this up in the corner of your room and turn it on when you're hanging with a girl. The laser will light up across the ceiling and the wall and create a cool, intimate atmosphere. It sets the mood immediately (it's been tested).

For this, I use this **LED Disco Ball**. It's never steered me wrong, and I highly recommend it (and yes, that's also me dancing in that video and dragging that girl across the dance floor at the beginning :p ...).

Element #4: Preparedness

Here's an element you might not have thought of, but trust me, it's important. And you're about to see why...

Have Your Condoms Ready

You're about to have sex with her. She's lying on your bed, ready for you to give her an amazing experience. Excitedly, you get up to grab a condom. Unfortunately, you can't remember where you put your stash. You search through a few drawers and closets and come up empty.

If this has ever happened to you, you know how much of a mood killer it is. And it sucks, especially because you can avoid it so easily.

That's why you need to come prepared (no pun intended, but intended).

You should have a condom in your wallet as well as a designated drawer/place in your room where you put your condoms. If you want to be extra prepared, you can put a condom under each pillow, too.

Sometimes, in the heat of the moment, and especially if you're drunk, it's easy to be irresponsible and go in without a condom. But if you have condoms under the pillows, you can beat your monkey brain and avoid the condomless sex you'll regret later.

Have Multi-Purpose Lubrication

We'll talk about sexual massages in the foreplay fundamentals – they're great for turning women on and teasing them before sex.

But a necessary part of those massages is massage lubrication. So make sure to have some handy in your drawer.

Look for a water-based massage lubricant that can double as sexual lube (KY has a few like this).

Because when you're giving her a sexual massage,

some of it is bound to eventually get between her legs, and it can make her feel a burning sensation if the massage lubrication isn't water-based, which can make sex painful later on, too.

Aside from this, sex lube is great because even if a woman is turned on, she can start to dry out after multiple sex sessions (or one particularly long session). The lube gets her wet again and allows the fun to keep going.

Stock Up on Wine/Liquor/Beer

As a general rule, you should always be stocked with:

- 1 bottle of red wine

- 1 bottle of liquor (vodka is a safe bet)

- 1-2 mixers

- 2 beers

There are two reasons for this.

1) You can use these as a way to bring her home (e.g. "Let's head back to my place for a drink.")

2) They help set the mood once you're at your place.

The funny thing is, usually you won't even finish a glass of wine/beer/a drink before you start hooking up with her.

As a side note, you should offer her a glass of water along with a drink. A lot of times (especially if you've taken her home after a long night of dancing and partying), she won't even want a drink (even if she agreed to "go back to your place for a drink"). But it's good to have it there, just in case.

***

Okay – you now know everything you need to in order to set up a great sexual experience. So, it's time to get the actual "hook up" started.

That's where the foreplay begins and what the next part will be all about!

Part IV:
The Foreplay Fundamentals

What Is Foreplay, and Why Is It Necessary?

You sit down in a fancy five-star restaurant.

You gaze at the surroundings and take it all in. Elegant decorations, well-dressed people, soothing music, and the enticing scent of delicious food.

You've heard about this place for months, and you finally managed to get a reservation after some intense effort...

And now, it's time to sit down and enjoy an amazing meal.

You want it all, too. An appetizer to whet your appetite and get you excited for the big meal, a main course to dig into, and a dessert to wind down.

You look at your friends across the table and say, "This is going to be awesome!"

But then, the waiter approaches your group and gives you some unfortunate news...

"I'm sorry, folks, but we've just run out of all of our appetizers. We're only serving the main course and dessert."

Your mood quickly changes from excitement to anxious disbelief. This was supposed to be the full five-star restaurant experience. The build-up, the climax, and the wind-down...

But now, you won't have the build-up. Not even a few pieces of bread with butter. Nope – they're just going to bring out your hearty steak for the main course in 30 minutes.

How would you feel if this happened?

Probably pretty disappointed, right?

Now imagine that feeling multiplied by a hundred...

That's what it can feel like to a woman when you skip out on foreplay. It can make the sex worse for you, too.

According to a study by the Journal of Sex Research [1], both men and women crave about 18 minutes of foreplay before sex.

Foreplay adds to the build-up and gets both you and your girl more excited to actually have sex (and it helps separate your mind from the stress and constant thoughts that come up in everyday life).

Then, when you and your girl eventually orgasm, the orgasm is much more pleasurable and powerful than had you gone straight in.

What's more, foreplay gets your girl wet (i.e. it naturally lubricates her vagina), and this is essential to great sex.

Yet a lot of guys like to slap on a condom and go right for it at the first chance they get. And even if they try to incorporate foreplay, they do it horribly wrong.

So Part IV of this book is all about getting foreplay right – so she's piping hot and ready for some amazing sex (and so you are, too).

Reference:

1. Miller, S. A., & Byers, E. S. (2004). Actual and desired duration of foreplay and intercourse: Discordance and misperceptions within heterosexual couples. *The Journal of Sex Research,41*(3), 301-309. doi:10.1080/00224490409552237

Fundamental #9: Know Her Most Important Parts

Most guys don't know the first thing about a woman's vagina. So it's no surprise that they have no idea what to do with it.

This isn't an anatomy text book, and you don't really need to know all of the parts of her vagina if you want to please her.

But it does help to know some of the most important parts, especially because I'll be referencing them throughout the rest of the book.

Don't get too caught up in memorizing all of these right now. Just make a mental note and know that you can refer back to this chapter if I reference a part that you don't understand.

The Mons Pubis

This is the skin just above the top of the vagina. It's a sensitive area and you can use this to tease a woman before you go all the way down to her vagina.

The Labia Minora and Labia Majora

These are the inner and outer lips of the labia. The labia is what you probably think of as the vagina. Everything kind of happens between these two lips, and they are very pleasurable for the woman.

The Clitoral Hood

The clitoral hood lies at the top of the labia majora, right above the clitoris.

Its purpose is to protect the clitoris because, as you're about to discover, it's very sensitive. It retracts into the skin as a woman moves closer to orgasm and reemerges from the hood after orgasm.

The Clitoris

Some even go so far as to call this the "female penis." Why? Well, it's filled with nerve endings and gets firmer and larger as the girl gets more stimulated. However, it's much smaller than the penis (which is why some guys struggle to find it), and it's used solely for sexual stimulation.

It's also known simply as "the clit." Keep in mind that some clits are bigger than others. It can be a little longer than an inch in length (though it's usually smaller than that), with a circumference somewhere between .1 and .3 inches. But that's just the part you see on the outside. The clit is like an iceberg — approximately 3 quarters of it are actually inside the body.

It's filled with around 8,000 nerve endings, which is more than anywhere else in the body and twice as many as are in the head of the penis. In other words, it's a tiny pleasure center for the woman.

You can find the clit just below the clitoral hood and just above the...

...The Vaginal Opening

This is the external opening to the vagina. It's where babies are born, and also where you actually put your penis (and fingers) into the woman.

The G Spot

This is a small patch of flesh located around 2-3 inches up inside the vagina on the front of the vaginal wall. It's an important area to hit when fingering her during foreplay.

The Anus

The anus is the external opening of the rectum. This isn't a part of the vagina (of course) but it can be a very pleasurable zone. Some women like when you lick their anus, and also when you put a finger inside of it when you're eating them out.

The Perineum

This is the small area of skin between the anus and the bottom of the vagina. It can be pleasurable to some women when you put a little pressure on it with your finger, while others won't feel much there.

***

Okay, you now have a better understanding of a woman's vagina than the majority of men. That's a good first step. But now, you need to put that information to use.

With this in mind, let's talk about how to get the physical part of foreplay going. We'll start with the art of the sexual massage.

Fundamental #10: Master the Art of the Sexual Massage

Have you ever wanted to give a woman a teasing erotic massage that makes her whole body burst with sexual energy – so she's practically begging you for sex?

Well, that's what this chapter is all about.

Now, you don't need to give a girl a sexual massage every time, but it's a powerful tool to have in your foreplay arsenal.

It adds variety and pleasure to the experience you have with a girl you've already been hooking up with (e.g. a girlfriend/fuck buddy/wife). Plus, it can lead a girl who was on the fence about having sex with you to basically give in and beg for your cock.

Most of all, it amplifies the sexual tension, turns her on, and gets her incredibly wet.

But before you get started giving sexual massages, you need to get the right tools. So let's start with that.

The Tools You'll Need to Give Her a Great Sexual Massage

I briefly mentioned these in the chapter about transforming your apartment into a panty-dropping bachelor pad, but I'll go more in-depth here (that way, you won't have to reference multiple chapters when you want to give her that sexy massage).

Scented Candles

Scented candles create a relaxed atmosphere with warm lighting and a pleasant aroma. Have three to four candles ready before you set up the massage and make sure to put them in a place where you won't knock them over during it (or during sex later). You don't want to burn the whole house down.

Experiment with different scents to see which you and your girl like best.

And make sure to have a lighter or some matches handy in your room so you don't have to scramble when you want to get the candles set up.

Incense

I hadn't used incense until recently when a roommate of mine told me about it. But I've been using it ever since. And it complements the scented candles well during the massage.

In addition to creating a subtle and pleasant scent in the room, incense can also stimulate sexual desire and increase sexual attraction.

Massage Oil

You need some lubrication for the massage – otherwise, it will be rough and potentially painful for the girl. So make sure to have some handy in your drawer.

As I mentioned earlier, go for a water-based massage lubricant that can double as sexual lube (KY has a few like this).

Because when you're giving her a sexual massage, some of it is bound to eventually get between her legs, and it can make her feel a burning sensation if the massage oil isn't water-based, which can make sex painful later on (I've had this happen before, and it's a mood killer).

Good Music

Relaxing, chill music sets the mood for a good sexual massage.

Again, I recommend the "Chill Vibes" playlist on Spotify. If you want to get fancy with it and add a little variation, you can try a more "spa" type of playlist, like the "Spa Music" one (this is less repetitive) on Spotify. It's super chill and also sets the mood well.

Start the Massage

Important note: Ask her what she likes in a massage and listen intently to her answer. The instructions I'll lay out are a great guide, but nothing beats specific instructions from the girl. A lot of girls know what they want in a massage, and you'll do just fine by giving it to them the way they like it.

Tell her to lie on her stomach and keep her underwear on (this is more subtle and better than telling her to strip down and take her clothes off).

Then start playing the music, light the candles and incense, and break out the massage oil. Take your shirt off as well. It's time to start the massage.

Position yourself so that you straddle her just below her butt (just make sure to hold your own weight so she can be comfortable). This gives you access to her whole back and butt, and it's also a sexual position. If you start to get hard (which you probably will at some point during the massage), she'll feel it around her anus and towards the bottom of her vagina, and it'll turn her on even more.

Once you're in position, pour the massage oil/lubricant onto your hands and start working her middle to upper back and shoulders (try and do it to the rhythm of the music – this will add to the experience for her). Do this for five to ten minutes.

Here are some techniques to use while massaging her back and shoulders:

- Start with long up and down strokes on her back. For good strokes, keep your fingers together, your thumbs parallel, and your palms in full contact with the part of the body that you're working.

- Don't forget about her arms and hands. You should also occasionally stroke the backs of her arms and caress her hands.

- Use compression. Lay one hand flat on her back, neck, or shoulder, and press the other hand on top of it. Rotate slowly and add a little pressure.

- Look for knots in her back and try to loosen them up by adding pressure.

Once you've done this for five to ten minutes, start gradually working down to her lower back and legs, all the way down to her feet.

From here, you can start making it more sexual...

Make It Sexual

At this point, she should be turned on quite a bit. If not, this will do the trick.

Work your hands slowly up one leg, with one hand on the inside and one on the outside. Turn your hands away from her pussy at the last moment, and instead slide them up closer to her ass. Then repeat with the other leg.

Now, run one hand up each of her legs simultaneously and again, move them away from her pussy at the last moment.

Repeat this process a few times, and she'll be very turned on. She might even start moaning.

Run your hands up her legs one more time, then start working her ass and lower back again and move to her upper back and shoulders. Lie across her back with your face near hers and remember to hold your own weight.

From there, gently pull her face closer to you from behind, turn her head slightly, and start kissing her neck and then her lips.

You can then turn her over and massage the front of her body or simply kiss her and her body and transition into foreplay (or sex). Either one works well.

Wrapping Up the Art of the Sexual Massage...

Once you give a girl a sexual massage, the mood should be very ON. She should be craving sex at this point even if the two of you haven't yet slept together.

To recap, here are the three important elements of the sexual massage:

- Get the right tools, like scented candles, incense, massage oil, and good music.

- Start the massage on her middle to upper back, shoulders, arms, and hands.

- Make the massage sexual by stroking her legs and turning away from her pussy at the last moment.

Fundamental #11: The "Finger Dance" That Makes Her Squirt

Your fingers are powerful when it comes to foreplay…

The problem is, most guys don't know the right way to use them. They jam their fingers in and just kind of hope for the best.

The result? Sometimes the guy gets lucky and hits the right spots. But usually, he leaves the girl wondering what the hell he's trying to accomplish down there, and sometimes he even hurts or scratches her by accident.

I'll show you a better approach so that you can turn girls on and give them orgasms just by using your hands.

But before we get into it, let's lay out a few ground rules…

Keep your hands well groomed.

You don't want to go down there with hands looking like Wolverine's or Freddy Krueger's. That's how you end up hurting a girl.

Instead, make sure to keep your hands and nails well groomed.

That means keep your finger nails trimmed and clean (no dirt underneath), and wash your hands consistently. This helps prevent the spread of bacteria and also helps you avoid accidental scratches and bleeding.

Tease her beforehand to get her wet and build anticipation.

It's much better to start fingering her when she's already wet and turned on than to go in there when she's dry.

This builds anticipation, which makes the experience better for her when you start fingering her.

So make sure to tease her beforehand. We'll talk more about that in the next fundamental, but here are a few tips:

- Give her a sexual massage like we talked about in the last chapter.

- Kiss her neck, ears, abdomen, and inner thighs.

- Give her sexual kisses on the lips.

Get comfortable.

Position yourself comfortably before you start fingering her. That way, you won't tire yourself out, and you can keep at it for as long as you need to.

Experiment with different positions to get a sense of which ones work best for you. For example, you can lie next to her and kiss her while doing it or get down in between her legs and do it from there.

Start slow.

Her vagina and clitoris are sensitive, so don't jam your fingers in and start flicking her clit at full force.

Start slow – graze her vagina and clit with your fingertips and create more build up.

Then insert the first finger and finger her slowly for a minute or two. Afterwards, add in the second finger and start revving things up.

Be aware of her reaction.

Like most things in sex, her reaction says it all. If she's moaning loudly hand seems to be enjoying herself, then keep doing what you're doing. She may be close to having an orgasm, and you shouldn't switch things up in that moment.

Have some lube ready.

You won't necessarily have to use it, especially if you get her really wet beforehand. But it's good to have nearby, just in case.

And if you go for multiple rounds of sex, the lube will make things easier, as she may dry out more quickly (even if she's turned on).

Okay, with those things in mind, let's get into the techniques…

The "Finger Dance" That Makes Her Squirt

There's a simple fingering method that can make most women squirt.

I remember when I first learned it…

I was living in Ho Chi Minh City, Vietnam, and I met an incredibly sexual Spanish girl.

She had a vibrant sexual energy that you could sense just by looking into her eyes. She was 10 years older than me and knew her way around the bedroom.

And she wasn't afraid to bluntly tell me what she liked and didn't like…

One night, as we were lying in bed, she turned to me…

"I want to show you something. This is the secret to making any girl squirt in minutes. And I want you to do it to me…"

I'd never made a girl squirt before, but I'd heard stories of it happening and seen it in porn. I'd always wanted to do it, and I knew this was my chance.

That's when she showed me the "finger dance" that I'm about to show you…

First, though, I should tell you that you don't need to do this every time. I break it out on occasion with a girl I really like. It's an intense experience, and I don't want to share it with just any girl – especially because it can create a powerful emotional response from her that you don't want unless you do indeed really like a girl.

Also, a couple of notes on squirting:

- Squirting is basically female ejaculation. It doesn't happen every time a girl has an orgasm, but it can happen occasionally during sex and fingering.

- When it happens, liquid literally squirts out of her vagina with force.

- It doesn't necessarily mean the orgasm is any better than a normal orgasm, but it does allow you to provide the girl with a unique and pleasurable experience that she probably hasn't had before.

- You don't need to use this technique solely to make her squirt. You can also use it just to get her extra wet and lubricated before sex or cunnilingus.

Here's how to do it...

1. Have her lie on your bed face up with her legs open.

2. Get into a comfortable position. Try lying on her left side so that you're perpendicular to her body (i.e. your bodies form an "L" shape," and your head is near her stomach so that you can see her vagina.

3. Insert your index finger and find her "G" spot. As I mentioned earlier, her G spot is usually two to three inches up against the front of her vaginal wall (if it feels ribbed and textured, you're on the right track).

4. Stroke her G spot slowly with your index finger, as though using it to make a "come hither" gesture.

5. After two or three minutes, speed up the strokes and insert your middle finger.

6. Cup her clit with the palm of your hand, and pull your hand up and down as you finger her. This will stimulate both her clit and her G spot at the same time.

7. Keep this going for 10-15 minutes, speeding up and going full force as she's about to climax. Get into it yourself too, and coach her by saying things like,

"Yes baby, you're so sexy, push for me baby, I love watching you cum."

Note: The most important thing is to get into a good rhythm with her. Some girls squirt much faster than others, so while 10-15 minutes is a good benchmark, every girl is different.

When you do this, keep in mind that the more comfortable a girl is with you, the easier it will be for her to squirt.

And if she doesn't squirt, don't beat yourself up over it. It's still a great way to turn her on and lead into sex.

The Slider

This one is a lot simpler than the finger dance we just talked about. It's great for when you want to quickly stimulate her and get her wet before cunnilingus or sex.

Start by putting your middle and ring fingers on her mons pubis above her vagina. Then slide them down on either side of her labia. Continue until you reach the vaginal opening and insert your fingers. Repeat this process and increase the speed as she becomes more aroused.

Experiment!

Don't just stick to these techniques. The goal here

isn't to get you thinking technically every time you want to finger a girl.

Instead, it's to give you a basis to go off of so you have a place to get started.

Experiment on your own and get to know a girl's vagina with your hands. Get a sense for what she likes and doesn't like. Hell, you might even come up with some of your own finger moves in the process.

A Note on Going Down Under...

More girls than you'd think like at least a little bit of ass play.

Some women may ask you to put a finger in their anus while you give them cunnilingus or finger them. Others like it but won't come out and tell you they want it right away.

If you're into this kind of thing too, you can experiment with a girl by putting a finger on her perineum and applying a little bit of pressure. If she reacts positively, move your finger closer to her anus. If her reaction is still positive, you can go for it by putting one finger inside of it.

Wrapping Up Fingering Techniques...

Your fingers are powerful tools for giving a girl orgasms and making her squirt. But like any set of tools, you have to use them the right way in order to be effective.

Here's a recap of this fundamental:

- Keep the ground rules in mind, like having well-groomed hands, teasing her beforehand, and starting slow.

- The more comfortable a girl is with you, the easier it will be for her to squirt.

- The "finger dance" and the slider are two great techniques to keep in mind when fingering a girl.

- Experiment yourself to see what each girl likes best.

- Some girls like anal play – so keep that in mind if you're into that kind of thing, too.

Fundamental #12: The Casanova Guide to Cunnilingus

Oral sex – also known as cunnilingus (when it's performed on a woman) – is the key to really amazing foreplay.

But like many aspects of sex, most men don't know how to do it right. And so the majority of women experience bad oral sex. It's awkward, it hurts, or it's just plain mediocre, and they can barely feel it.

But if you can give your woman good cunnilingus, she'll love you for it. She'll want to have sex again and again, and you'll be able to please her with ease.

The funny thing is, it's not hard to give great cunnilingus if you know what to do. But again, most guys go in at random and hope for the best. They lap the girl's pussy up like a dog and use no finesse.

If you apply what you learn in this chapter, though, you'll put yourself ahead of the majority of men who never even consider how to improve their cunnilingus skills.

I'll start by showing you the right way to tease her, as this will get her revved up and make the cunnilingus exponentially more pleasurable for her. Then I'll give you some techniques you can use as well as the signs that tell you she's thoroughly enjoying what you're doing down there.

Let's get into it...

Tease Her (Don't Go for the Clit Right Away)

Foreplay is all about teasing, and even teasing has different levels. Cunnilingus is the last level – it's what all the rest of the foreplay builds up to.

So you shouldn't go right for clit – allow for some build-up first. Build the anticipation up to the point when she can barely handle it anymore, and then get started.

Here are some ways to tease her before you start the cunnilingus:

Kiss her erogenous zones.

Erogenous zones are areas of the body with heightened sensitivity. When you kiss and caress these zones, you'll instantly turn a woman on. Let's go through each of these zones:

- **Her ears.** Kiss and suck her ears, and nibble on her ear lobes.

- **Her neck.** Kiss, suck on, and gently bite her neck.

- **Her lips.** Give her sexual kisses and gently bite her lower lip.

- **Her breasts.** Caress her breasts by circling her nipples with your fingers. Kiss around the nipples, then gently start kissing and sucking on them.

- **Her inner thighs.** Start by running your hands down each of her inner thighs, then turn away right when you get close to her vagina. Then, starting from the top, kiss both of her inner thighs down to her ankles and back up again.

Give her a sexual massage.
Put what you learned from the sexual massage fundamental into action.

Kiss around her vagina.

After sucking on her breasts, slowly move down and kiss and lick her stomach. Right as you get to the mons pubis (the area just above her vagina), turn away and move to her inner thighs. You can lightly breathe on her vagina as you go down, which adds more intensity to the teasing.

And when you do make the move for her vagina, don't go for the clit right away. Kiss and lick her inner labia and the parts around the clit first.

Use your fingers.

Lightly graze her vagina and clit with your fingers after you kiss her erogenous zones.

***

Use at least a few of these tips to tease her, and she'll be ready to go for cunnilingus. Hell, she'll probably even be begging you to do it.

At that point, you can use some of the cunnilingus techniques below:

Cunnilingus Techniques That Will Drive Her Wild

Half the battle is knowing what to do – that way, you don't end up slobbering around her vagina without a purpose or clue.

Before we get into specific techniques, though, I'll give you some basics for good cunnilingus. If you follow these, you'll be able to perform any technique well.

- **Start slow.** Don't go in there with full force right from the outset. Start slow and gradually build up to make it more and more intense. This allows you to pace yourself as well so that you don't run out of steam and tire out your tongue too quickly.

- **Make occasional eye contact.** Just as you'll enjoy when a girl looks up at you when she gives you head, the girl will enjoy it when you return the favor. So look up at her and make eye contact occasionally as you perform cunnilingus – it makes the experience more intense and immersive.

- **Use the different parts of your tongue (with some force).** Your tongue is a muscle with different parts to it. So add some strength behind it when you eat her out.

- **Don't just rely on your tongue.** You can also rotate your head and jaw to add intensity and assist your tongue with the movements.

- **Moan and show her you like it.** As you'll learn in the next set of fundamentals, women like when you moan and grunt during sex and foreplay. When you moan during foreplay, it shows her that you enjoy what you're doing, and it reassures her that you're happy to be down there. This is key because some girls can be insecure about their lady parts.

- **Tongue movements.** Side to side, flicking, and circular motions on her clit with your tongue will drive her wild. When in doubt, move your tongue so that it hits different parts of her clit and labia.

- **Rhythm.** This is especially important when she's on her way to coming. You need to be able to maintain the rhythmic tongue motion and give her continued stimulation. If you stop when she's about to finish, you may rob her of an orgasm.

- **Fingers.** You don't always need to use your fingers during cunnilingus, but they can help. You can put one or two fingers in and finger her to the rhythm of your tongue motions. You can also just leave the finger in without moving it much.

Now that you know the basics, here are some tried and true cunnilingus techniques that you can use...

First, I'll note that you shouldn't get too caught up in whether or not you're doing the technique right. For example, don't think, "Am I making the right circles?!" Just keep them in the back of your mind as you do the basics. You'll know if she's enjoying it by the way she reacts (which you'll learn more about at the end of this chapter).

1) Circles

Position your tongue on the right or left side of her clit. Then move it around only the clit in a clockwise or counterclockwise motion.

This stimulates the clit from the outside of the hood and also allows you to make contact with the clit underneath the hood when you're at the 6 o'clock position.

You can vary this by starting softly with slow circles, then using more force and increasing speed as she gets closer to orgasm.

2) ABCs

You may have heard of this one before, and it may even seem like a joke, but it's actually a legitimately good technique.

Simply position your tongue on either side of her clit or at the top, and use your tongue to draw your ABCs.

This provides just the right amount of contact with both the clitoral hood and the clitoral head while adding lots of variation (since no two strokes are exactly the same).

And if you want to add even more variation to it, you can trace out words, sentences, and geometrical shapes.

(Geometry 101 will finally come in handy!)

3) Sweeping

Position your tongue on either the right or left side of her clit. Then move from side to side as if you were sweeping a floor.

You can vary between fast and slow strokes to maximize pleasure. You can also go with long vertical strokes instead of side-to-side strokes.

4) Tongue Penetration

This is a good way to switch things up and give her a unique sensation.

Use your tongue to thrust in and out of her vaginal opening a few times as your lips make contact with her inner labia.

5) Vacuum

Put your lips around her clit so that it's in your mouth and lightly suck it – similar to the way you'd suck through a straw but gentler. The gentleness is key because it'll make her uncomfortable if you suck on it too hard.

You can add variety to this by combining it with the circle technique. While the clit is in your mouth, lick it in a circular motion.

Signs She's Enjoying the Cunnilingus

The techniques and basics are great, but how do you know if she's actually enjoying the cunnilingus?

Here are some signs that she's loving the experience:

- **She moans.** While some girls are mostly silent with light moans when they like it, others will moan loudly. Pay attention to her moans – the more she does it, the closer she usually is to coming.

- **She holds your head down in her vagina with her hand.** This is a clear sign that she wants you to stay down there and keep doing what you're doing.

- **She bites her lip.** If she does this, then you're doing something right.

- **She's says, "Just like that."** Phrases like this tell you that you should keep doing exactly what you're doing. Not faster, not in a different rhythm, but the same thing.

How Long Should You Perform Cunnilingus?

There is no set amount of time for performing cunnilingus.

You can use it as a tool to make a girl orgasm. In this case, it can take anywhere from 5 to 20 minutes or more depending on the girl.

You can also use it as a tool to increase excitement and turn her on, which will lead to better sex. In this case, you can do it for as long as you want, but don't stop if you notice she's about to have an orgasm.

Wrapping Up the Casanova Guide to Cunnilingus...

If you can perform cunnilingus well, you'll drive women wild and make them crave sex with you. You'll also find it a lot easier to give women orgasms.

Here's a quick recap of the chapter:

- Tease her before the cunnilingus by kissing her

erogenous zones, giving her a sexual massage, using your fingers, and kissing around her vagina.

- Keep the cunnilingus basics in mind, like starting slow, hitting the clit from different angles, using different parts of your tongue, pacing yourself, and making occasional eye contact.

- Use techniques like circles, sweeping, and the vacuum to enhance the cunnilingus experience.

- Know the signs to look for when she's enjoying the cunnilingus.

- Don't stop too soon.

Fundamental #13: Teach Her to Give You Great Head (so She Gets Addicted)

For those not familiar with the slang, "giving head" is when a girl sucks your dick. It's a blowjob.

Not every girl gives great head, and that's a damn shame. I'd say probably about 30% of women give amazing blowjobs, 40% of women give average blowjobs, and 30% of women give mediocre blowjobs.

The women who do give great head seem to enjoy it and get turned on by it the most. In fact, I've seen women literally have orgasms from giving head. It's like they're addicted to it.

These particular women enjoy pleasing you so much that it gets them off to do so. They could literally give you head all day.

Of course, getting head turns you on as well, makes you harder, and gets you ready to fuck her the way she needs to be fucked.

So it's pretty damn key that a girl gives you great head.

But what do you do if your girl is average or below average at giving head?

You can teach her to give you great head!

When a girl goes from average or mediocre to great at giving head, she'll enjoy it more, get addicted to pleasing you, and want to do it all the time.

*(Credit to my man Christian McQueen of **https://realchristianmcqueen.com/** for some of these tips. I started doing this a lot more after I learned about it from him.)*

Here's How to Teach Her to Give You Great Head...

Sit on a chair and put a pillow in front of you. Tell her to get undressed and kneel on the pillow.

Tell her, "Baby, I want you to take your time giving me head, and I'll show you exactly what I like."

Walk her through it and tell her exactly what you want. For example:

- "Open your mouth wider"
- "Spit on it"
- "Jerk it with your hands for a few seconds"
- "Hold it with your hand while you suck on it"

- "Gag for me"
- "Choke on it"
- "Look up at me while you suck it"
- "Use more tongue"
- "No teeth."
- "Suck on my balls"

(It's important to do this in a dominant way – don't worry, you'll learn about this in Part V.)

After one or two times doing this, you should be able to take her from an average or below average head-giver to an amazing one. And both of your sex lives will be a lot better as a result.

155

Part V:
The Sex
Fundamentals

Fundamental #14: Consent and Protection

We're in the most fun section of the book – the part about actually having sex!

It's the part you've probably been waiting for all along (though hopefully you've read everything up until now – that'll be a big factor in deciding whether or not you can actually put the following fundamentals to good use).

But before we dive into the fun stuff, we need to talk about a couple of not-so-fun subjects...

Consent and protection. These are two things that you can't really avoid when it comes to talking about sex...

A Note on Consent

It should go without saying, but you should never try to have sex with a girl without her consent. Morally, it's messed up to take advantage of a woman and force her to have sex with you against her will. And legally, it can screw up your whole life.

A big reason that I hope you're reading this book is

to be able to give women an amazing sexual experience. Well, you can't do that if she doesn't want to have sex with you in the first place!

So, here's what this means...

If she's clearly drunk, don't have sex with her.

We've all seen the guy at the bar making out with the sloppy drunk girl. She can barely stand up, and she clearly isn't fully aware of what's going on. It's best to avoid women who are too drunk because not much good will come out of that situation. If you happen to meet a cool girl who suddenly gets a little too drunk at some point in the night (which happens from time to time), I suggest calling her a taxi home or bringing her back to her friends.

Keep an eye out for girls who slur their words as well. They might be able to compose themselves to a point, but they let out subtle signals that they're actually wasted.

Overall, there's a big difference between going on a date with a girl and having one or two drinks together, then bringing her home, and meeting a girl at the club who is already five to ten drinks deep.

What's more, it's a big red flag when a girl goes out and gets hammered on a consistent basis. It's best to stay away from this type of girl in general, as she's bound to get you into some bad situations (or cheat on you if you end up dating her).

The hard "no."

You're hooking up with a girl in bed, clothes start coming off, and then all of a sudden she gives you the hard "no" (i.e. she says "no" in a somewhat serious tone).

As in, "No, I don't want to have sex with you."

When you get it, it's pretty clear that the girl does not want to have sex. At least, not that night.

(Note: This is different from when a girl says something like, "You know we're not going to have sex tonight, right?" before she comes back to your place. That's token resistance, and she's only saying it so she doesn't feel like a slut for going back with you. If I had a dollar for every time a girl said that and then wound up begging me to fuck her an hour later, I'd be a rich man.)

If you get this hard "no," pull back right away (even if you're in the middle of having sex with her). Either leave her place, or offer to call her a taxi home if she's at your place.

Sometimes these women can change their minds and then want to have sex later in the night, but it's not worth the risk, and it's also a big red flag. It's best to move on to a girl who is more open to sex with you.

How to get consent without being awkward...

Consent can be kind of a weird line because most times the girl won't say, "Yes, please put your penis inside of me." She might say, "You should get a condom..." and that should tell you that the answer is yes.

Or you can say, "I'm going to get a condom..." She may nod her head, or she may just not give any response. In the latter case, you can just say something like, "Cool?"

If she nods her head and/or says yes, then you've got consent.

Whatever the case, always get some type of verbal and/or nonverbal agreement that she's cool with having sex.

A Note on Protection

Yes, you should always use protection – even if you know a girl well and have been hanging with her for a while. The one exception is perhaps if you're in an exclusive relationship with a girl, AND she's on birth control. But even then, you still shouldn't finish inside her (unless you like the idea of some little babies running around in 9 months).

Why? The risks are obvious...

Unplanned pregnancy and STDs – two things that can

turn your life upside down real quick.

With that in mind, you'll need condoms. But what I've found is the type of condom you use can have a huge impact on the quality of sex.

Some condoms just don't have enough lubrication and will dry out too quickly (even if the girl is really wet), while others are too thin and have a tendency to break (and that's never fun).

Others are too thick and ruin the feeling completely.

So, how do you find the right condom for you?

Experiment with different types of condoms – buy a few three-packs and see which you like the most.

My favorite condom by far is the Trojan Fire & Ice condom. I started using these a couple years ago, and I've never turned back. If you haven't tried these out yet, I highly recommend giving them a shot.

Overall, I highly recommend the Trojan condom brand over any other condom brand... by far.

I've lived in several countries that don't sell Trojan condoms, and I always make sure to bring a stock of Trojans along with me.

I'm not affiliated with Trojan... I'm just a dude who has a lot of sex and can appreciate a good condom (and who is also sick of shitty and tiny condoms that squeeze the life out of me).

***

Okay, we've covered the tough stuff. Now it's time to get to the more fun stuff!

In the next chapter, we'll talk about the best sex positions. So get ready...

Fundamental #15: 10 Orgasmic Sex Positions to Drive Her Wild (and How to Use Them)

You should have some good sex positions in your arsenal.

The positions themselves won't make sex great. The way you use them will.

The rhythm with which you put them into practice, the dominance you convey when you move her into these positions, and the degree to which you vary the positions. These will all have a bigger impact on the quality of sex than the positions themselves (and you will learn about all of these things in this part of the book).

Some men, for example, try a bunch of different positions throughout their sex sessions with women, but they never get the rhythm down, and so the sex isn't good. Other men use the positions well, but they try to do too much and tire themselves out quickly.

My point is, sex positions are important. But they are not the be-all and end-all. You can't rely solely on them and expect to have great sex.

But when you combine great sex positions with the other fundamentals we've talked about (and will talk about throughout the rest of this book), you can transform a sex session from average to amazing.

You can use the positions to help you last longer (both in terms of your stamina and your ability to control your orgasm), connect deeply with the girl, add variety, and stimulate important parts of her body.

So keep that in mind as you go through this chapter.

Here are a few more important notes before I show you the positions...

Don't be so quick to switch things up. If you switch positions every minute or two, you'll have a tough time getting into a sexual rhythm with a girl, and she'll have a tougher time reaching orgasm. It's better to stay in a position until you get the urge to switch things up, usually after five to ten minutes (sometimes longer) or until the girl signals that she wants to switch things up.

Skin-to-skin contact. Some of these positions maximize skin-to-skin contact, which adds more intimacy and pleasure to the experience and can also give you the bonus of stimulating her clit as you thrust. On the other hand, some of these positions minimize skin-to-skin contact, which allows you to be more dominant and adds variety to the experience. You should have a good mix of positions both with and without a lot of skin-to-skin contact.

Keep your sexual stamina in mind. Some positions will give you a lot of stimulation and might cause you to lose control and come quickly. If you feel this happening before you want to come, then switch positions to one with less stimulation. For example, you could switch from *scissor doggy style* to *missionary with full contact*. On the other hand, some positions will tire you out more quickly. If you feel this happening, then switch to a position where you don't have to expend as much energy. For example, you could switch from *mirror doggy style* to *her on top*.

You can use the same position multiple times. Sex positions aren't like baseball pitchers or the Cleveland Browns' quarterbacks. Once you stop using one, you don't have to toss it out for the rest of the session. You can go back to it multiple times. For example, I typically use *missionary with full contact*, *lying flat doggy style*, and *her on top* multiple times during a sex session. These are kind of like my "default positions." I like them because they're pleasurable and also make it easy to transition to a number of other, different positions.

There are other positions, too. There are hundreds, if not thousands, of different sex positions, but these are some of the most powerful and pleasurable. I came across several of these through experimentation, while I heard about others (or saw them in porn) and tried them myself, then added my own variations. So, don't get caught up in thinking these are your only sex position options. Try them out and see which you like and which work well. Experiment, add variations, and hell, you might just come up with your own awesome new sex position. It's all part of the fun.

Be aware of when she's about to come. One of the biggest mistakes you can make is to abruptly switch positions when a girl is about to have an orgasm. If you notice her moaning more intensely, breathing hard, or if she straight up tells you she's about to come, then don't switch positions! If you do, you'll most likely rob her of her orgasm. However, a lot of guys —especially when they're new to sex – will start to lose control when she's about to come. In the case that you feel like you're losing control, it's better to switch positions so that you don't come too early, even if it means that she doesn't ride that wave and achieve orgasm at that moment. This helps you avoid coming too early before she comes, which will be a big downer. You can always get back into a rhythm again once you're used to the stimulus. As a good friend of mine likes to say, "I'd rather go slow for ten minutes so I can fuck for thirty more."

Now, with this in mind, let's get into the actual sex positions!

I'll score each one based on the level of skin-to-skin contact, the energy you'll have to use to do it, the variations it has (if any), and the easiest position to transition to afterwards. I'll also include an illustration for each position so you can visualize it.

*(To see all of these illustrations handbook-style online, go to: **http://bit.ly/10-positions**)*

1. Missionary With Full Contact

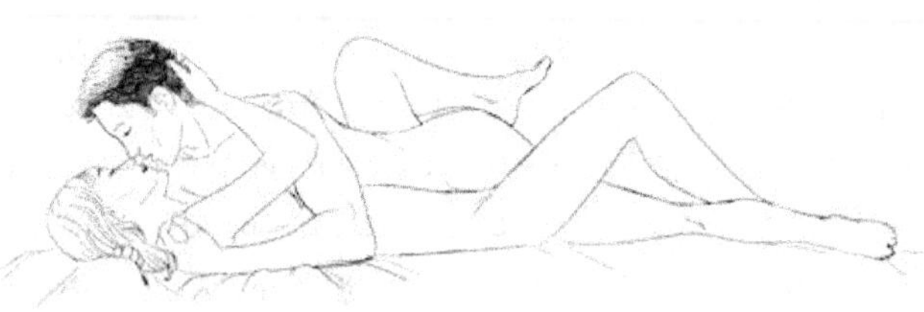

Skin-to-skin contact: *Maximized*

Energy used: *Medium*

This isn't your traditional "awkward sex on prom night" missionary position. You know, the one with your arms on either side of the girl, hoisting yourself up above her while you pump in and out.

No, this is the evolved (and much more pleasurable) version.

This is one of the best (if not *the* best) position to start with. It's simple, allows you to get a good rhythm going, and doesn't expend too much of your energy too quickly. It also allows you to control the pace so you don't overstimulate yourself and come before you want to.

Here's how to do it...

While she's on her back, get on top of her and position yourself in between her legs like you'd normally do with missionary.

But, instead of hoisting yourself up with your hands, position your body against hers so that your torsos rub against each other. Put both elbows and forearms on the bed up near her shoulders for support.

Place your left hand behind her neck and your right hand behind her left shoulder. This will help you get more leverage for thrusting and also make it easy to grab the roots of her hair in a dominant way (we'll talk more about that later in this part of the book).

Why is this position great? Aside from the fact that it helps you set the rhythm and get things off to a good start, it also maximizes contact between her clitoris and your pelvic region. This combination of vaginal and clitoral stimulation can lead to a quick orgasm or, at the very least, a lot of added pleasure for the girl.

Best position to transition to: *Scissor doggy style*

Variations:

- Wrap her legs around your waist.

- Grab both of her ass cheeks with your hands and use them to pull yourself into her on each thrust.

- Lift her by her lower back with both hands, hoist her up gently, and thrust (keep in mind this expends a lot more energy on your part).

- While holding her head by the root of her hair with one hand, place the other hand on her butt cheek. This allows you to grab her ass and also stroke her leg and upper thigh.

- Put a pillow underneath her butt to help get a better angle.

- Kiss her neck and nibble on her ear while you penetrate her.

2. Scissor Doggy Style

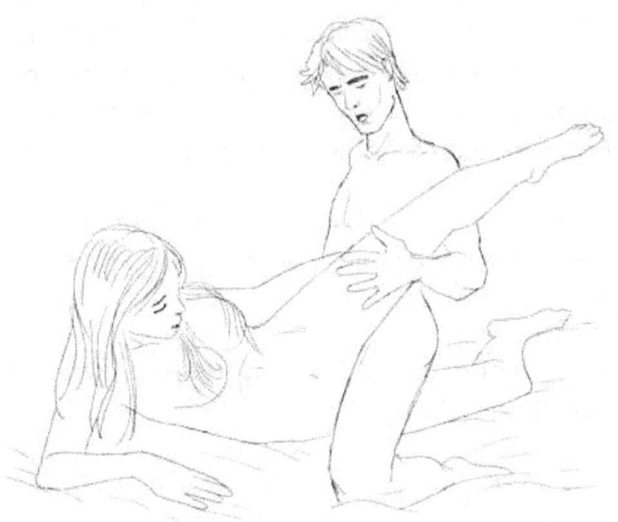

Skin-to-skin contact: *Medium*

Energy used: *Medium*

This is pretty much the "go-to" position I transition to after *missionary with full contact*. I think it's a slightly rarer position based on the pleasantly surprised looks I get from girls when I do it. I've also had several girls tell me they'd never even seen a guy try it before.

Here's how to do it...

If you're already fucking her in the *missionary with full contact* position, then you don't even need to take your penis out of her vagina.

Sit up on your knees and turn her onto her right side with both of her legs together (if you're familiar with yoga, this looks like the sideways savasana pose where she's lying down on her side with both her legs curled up together to one side).

Then, lift her inner leg (i.e. the one not touching the bed), and move your body forward so that her outer leg is between your knees.

At this point, you're basically sitting up straight with her right leg inside the gap between your legs.

This allows you to thrust deeply and easily grab her ass and titties.

Best position to transition to: *Doggy style*

Variation: *Instead of getting in between her legs, fuck her while both of her legs are together and you're kneeling behind them. Here, you're fucking her while she's in the "savasana" type of pose that I just mentioned.*

3. Doggy Style

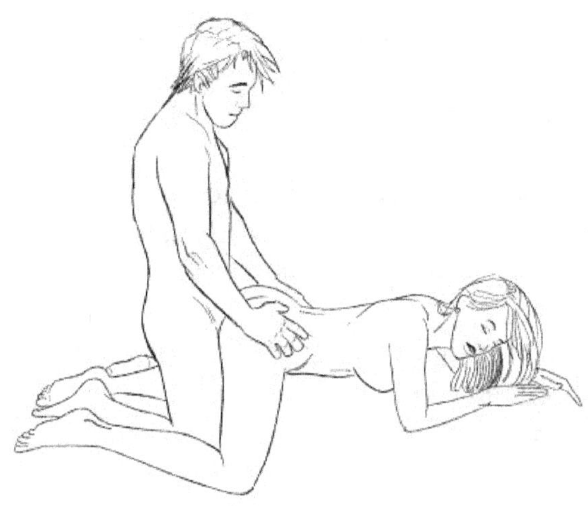

It's the tried-and-true position that you've almost certainly heard of already.

It gives you a great view of her ass and body and easy access to spanking her.

What I've noticed is that the better a girl's ass is, the more likely she's going to want to get into this position first. She'll hop on the bed and hoist her ass up. So hop on there and give her what she wants!

Here's how to do it:

Have her get on the bed on all fours. Get up behind her while you're on your knees and start thrusting.

Reach around and occasionally grab her titties. You can also reach around and rub her clit with your fingers, since the position itself doesn't stimulate it.

Best position to transition to: *Lying flat doggy style*

Variations:

- Sit back so that your butt touches your ankles, and pull her ass and upper body back so that her back touches your chest while you enter her from behind.

- Put one leg up near her side like you're taking a knee, and continue thrusting. This will help you thrust deeper.

4. Lying Flat Doggy Style

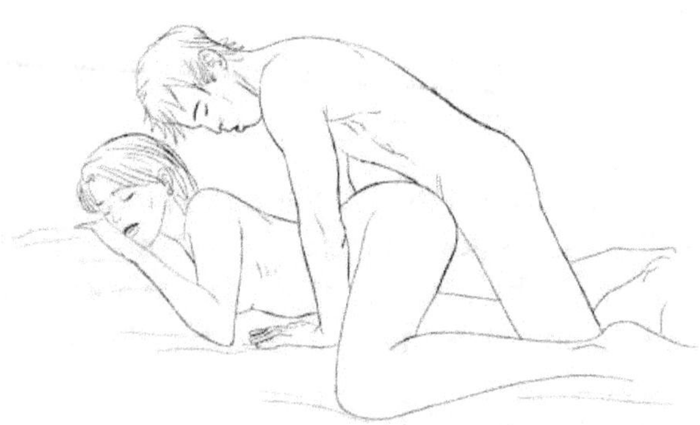

Skin-to-skin contact: *Medium to maximum*

Energy used: *Medium to high*

This position gives you a lot of what's awesome about regular doggy style but adds more skin-to-skin contact.

Here's how to do it...

Have her get into the regular doggy style position and penetrate her. Then have her lie flat down on the bed with her legs together. Get on top of her so that your stomach is touching her back. Start thrusting.

This allows you to easily kiss her neck from behind, talk dirty into her ear, and spank her.

Best position to transition to: *Doggy style*

Variations:

- *While inside of her, turn your body so that it's perpendicular to hers and keep thrusting.*

- *Instead of thrusting, have her rotate her ass so that she's controlling the speed and type of penetration.*

- *Put a pillow under her lower abdomen to get in at a better angle.*

5. Her on Top

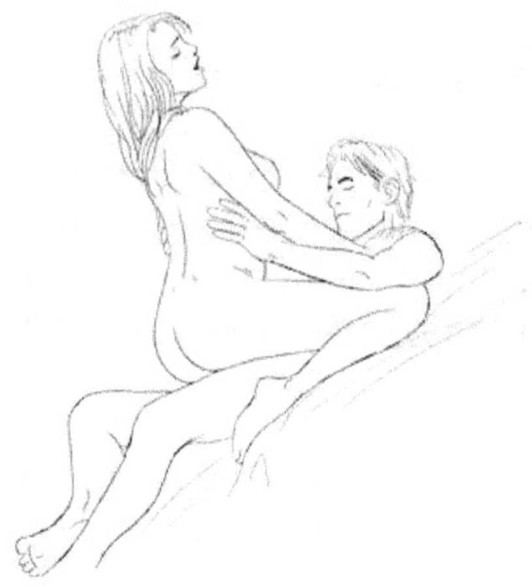

Skin-to-skin contact: *Low to medium*

Energy used: *Low*

Here's another classic position.

Her on top can be intimate or rough. She can do most (or all) of the work, or you can switch it up, grab her ass, and thrust into her.

Here's how to do it...

Lie down on the bed and tell her to get on top and ride you.

While she rides you, you can grab her titties, ass, and whatever part of her body you want. Enjoy the view and watch those titties bounce up and down as she pleasures the both of you.

Best position to transition to: *Reverse cowgirl*

Variations:

- *Put your knees up, bring her in closer to you, and thrust into her.*

- *Hoist yourself up so that your torso is parallel to hers, and suck on her titties.*

- *Move to the edge of the bed and put your feet on the floor. Have her straddle you while she faces you. This dramatically increases skin-to-skin contact and allows you to go deeper.*

6. Reverse Cowgirl

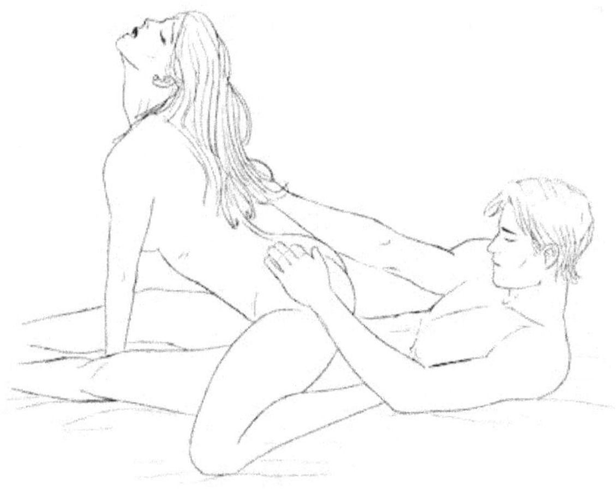

Skin-to-skin contact: *Low*

Energy used: *Low*

This is basically the reverse of her on top. It gives you a clear view of her ass as she rides you while facing in the opposite direction.

Here's how to do it...

Lie down on the bed and position her so that her ass is facing you, and she's looking towards your feet. Tell her to ride you.

Smack her ass and enjoy the view as she goes up and down.

Best position to transition to: *Edge-of-bed reverse cowgirl*

Variation: *Bring her lower back towards you, bend your knees, and thrust into her.*

7. Edge-of-Bed Reverse Cowgirl

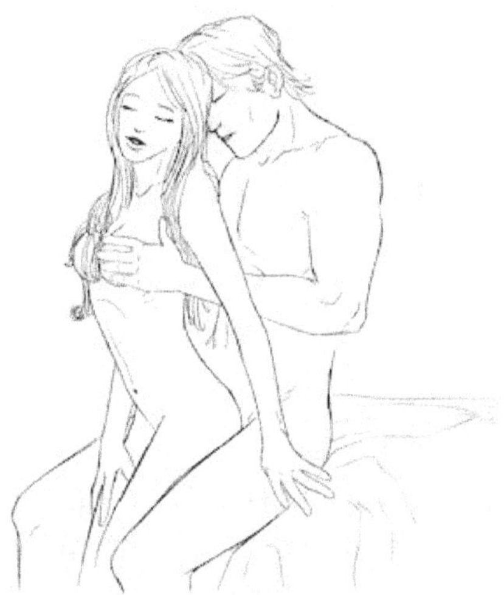

Skin-to-skin contact: *Low to medium*

Energy used: *Low*

This one is similar to regular reverse cowgirl in that she's riding you while facing in the opposite direction.

But instead of lying down, you're on the edge of the bed with your feet on the floor. It's great for making more skin-to-skin contact

Here's how to do it...

Sit on the edge of the bed so that your feet are

planted on the ground. Spread your legs apart a bit so that she can easily sit on you and put her own legs between them. Then, position her so that she can ride you with both of her legs together and her ass facing you. Her feet should be touching the ground too.

It's basically like how you'd imagine a lap dance, except instead of dancing on you, she's fucking you.

Best position to transition to: *Mirror (or Standing) Doggy Style*

Variations:

- *Wrap your arms around her lower waist and move her up and down as you thrust into her.*

- *Lie back like you would during regular reverse cowgirl.*

8. Mirror (or Standing) Doggy Style

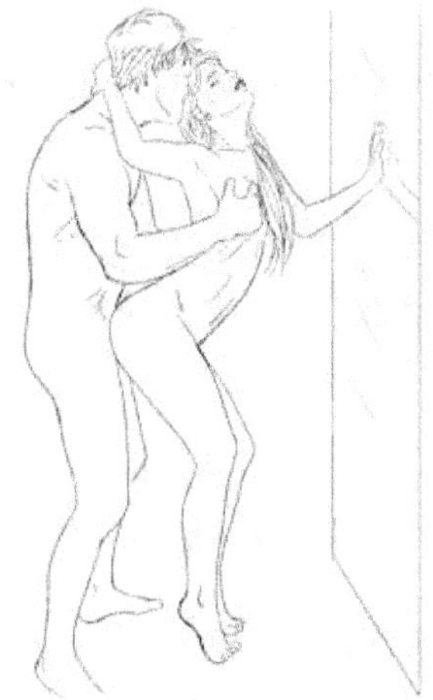

Skin-to-skin contact: *Low to Medium*

Energy used: *High*

This is the standing up version of doggy, except it's enhanced with the help of a mirror.

(All the better if you have a big mirror near your bed so that you can do this easily.)

The mirror is great because it allows you to see each other's expressions and full bodies. You can see her moan and watch her titties bounce, and she can see the pleasure that she's giving you.

Here's how to do it...

Tell her to stand up and plant her hands near (or on)

the mirror (either on the wall, the bureau, or something else that's sturdy).

Then, thrust into her vagina from behind.

You can wrap your arms around her waist, grab her titties for leverage, and even yank her head up by the root of her hair so that she looks in the mirror and watches as you fuck her.

Best position to transition to: *Any doggy style position, as well as edge-of-bed reverse cowgirl*

Variation: *Turn so that the sides of your bodies are facing the mirror instead of looking at it head on. That way, you can see the sex from a different angle and intensify the experience.*

9. Legs Over Shoulders

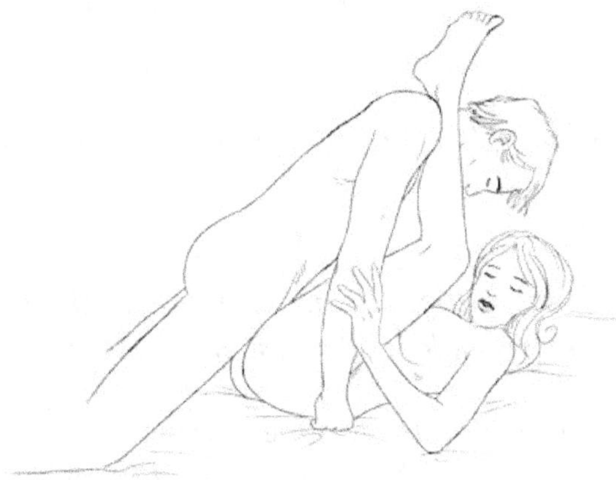

Skin-to-skin contact: *Medium*

Energy used: *High*

This is a little tweaking of the missionary position that allows you to go deeper and enjoy the feeling of her beautiful legs.

Just be careful not to go too deep here as this can hurt her.

Here's how to do it...

Have her lie down on the bed. Get between her legs and raise them as you thrust into her. Lean forward so that your face is above her breasts (or above her face if she's on the shorter side, or you're on the taller side), and her legs are straddling your shoulders.

Thrust in and out and enjoy the view of her entire upper body.

Best position to transition to: *Scissor doggy style*

Variations:

- Hold her legs straight up and together slightly to your left or right side, and continue thrusting.

- Stand on the floor at the edge of the bed. Pull her in so that her ass is on the edge, then put her feet over your shoulders and thrust. This gives you a little more thrusting power than when you're on your knees on the bed.

10. Her on Top (While You're Sitting on a Chair)

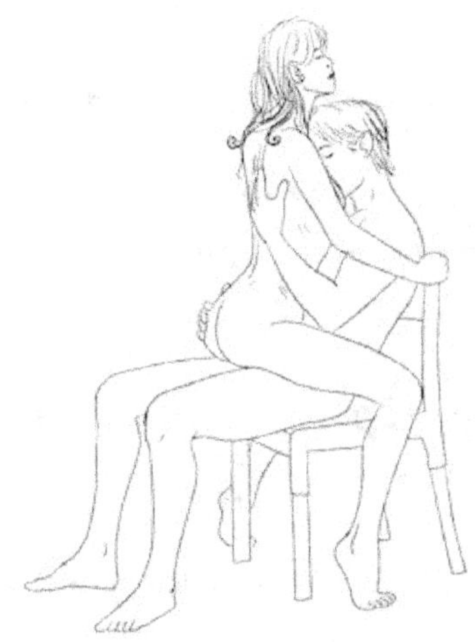

Skin-to-skin contact: *High*

Energy used: *Low to medium*

If you have a somewhat narrow chair with no arm rests, this one is the perfect way to utilize it.

Sit down on the chair and have her straddle you so that her legs are on either side of you.

Have her ride you up and down and side to side.

You can grab her ass and help her move in whatever way you want her to ride you.

This position allows you to get deeper and also make direct contact with the clitoris.

Best position to transition to: *Reverse cowgirl*

Variation: *Wrap your arms around her lower waist and suck on her titties while you help hoist her up and down or back and forth.*

Wrapping Up the Sex Positions (and How to Use Them)...

You've now got plenty of sex positions in your arsenal. You know how to transition between them, how to add variety to them, and how to make them more intense.

The rest of the sex fundamentals we'll cover will allow you to make the most out of every one of these positions and give her an experience quite unlike any she's ever had before.

To recap, here are the positions:

1. Missionary with full contact

2. Scissor doggy style

3. Doggy style

4. Lying flat doggy style

5. Her on top

6. Reverse cowgirl

7. Edge-of-bed reverse cowgirl

8. Mirror (or standing) doggy style

9. Legs over shoulders

10. Her on top while you're sitting on a chair

Fundamental #16: Dominance (The Right Way to Have Rough Sex)

If you forced me to choose the most important fundamental in this book, it'd be this one.

Dominance is perhaps the biggest key when it comes to having mind-blowing sex with a woman. Without it, you won't be able to get her off consistently.

You see, the feminine loves to be dominated. That's why women love men who dominate their own lives and go for what they want. That's why they love books like *50 Shades of Grey*.

But most men don't know how to dominate women in the bedroom. They're more vanilla than soft serve ice cream.

Here are some non-dominant things that most vanilla men do in the bedroom:

- **They ask, "Did you like it?"** They crave validation from women and just want to get a nod saying that they did an okay job.

- **They ask, "Is this good for you?"** They don't have the sexual awareness or confidence to be sure whether a girl likes something or not.

- **They ask instead of command.** "Can you give me a blowjob?" "Can we have sex doggy style?" "Can I come on your tits?" These men are always asking permission instead of taking what they want. This is a big turn-off for women.

- **They avoid rough sex.** The average guy doesn't want to have rough sex because he's afraid the girl won't like it. So he sticks mostly with regular missionary, pushing himself up above the girl and looking into her eyes as he gingerly pumps away.

All of this probably sounds a bit... weak, right? It should.

(I'm guessing you've probably never heard a girl say, "The sex was amazing! He was so kind the whole time. He asked permission before we switched positions, made sure I was enjoying it, and he even thanked me afterwards! What a gentleman!")

Men like this are the ones who complain that their women hardly ever want to have sex anymore. They're the men whose women run off with guys that know how to fuck a girl well (you know, the types of guys that read this book and take action on it).

You must not be like these non-dominant, weak

men. If you want to have mind-blowing sex with women, you must make a shift.

*(**Note:** If you see yourself as a non-dominant guy right now, don't sweat it. I used to be that way too. The beautiful thing is that you can transform into a more dominant man, and it starts with following the advice in this book, and especially within this chapter. So, keep an open mind as you read, and you will avoid the fate of the many weak-minded men of the world!)*

Here's the thing you need to realize: Women are not all the innocent little good girls that society would have you believe. They want to be fucked hard, manhandled, and dominated. And this is especially true for women with a lot of career success that are used to being in the leadership role. Many of these women are turned on by losing control and having a man take them in a dominant way - they often like it even harder.

So now you might be wondering, "How can I be more dominant?"

I'll give you a variety of ways to do so in this chapter. If you've never done any of them before, I recommend you start slow and gradually include more of these things in your sex sessions.

Some of these things may seem a bit extreme to you. But an overwhelming majority of women love all of this dominant behavior, and they'll orgasm a lot harder when you do it.

Here are some ways you can be dominant in the bedroom...

*(**Note:** Have a little caution with this stuff the first time you have sex with a girl. For example, she might like to get her hair pulled a little bit but dislike getting spanked. If you try something a little bit and can sense she likes it, you can keep upping the level. You can also talk about what kind of stuff she loves to do in bed after you've had sex and do it in the next session.)*

Give Her Commands

Stop asking permission during sex. If a woman doesn't like something, she'll let you know, either with her words or facial expressions.

Instead of asking her permission, give her commands. By giving her commands, you allow her to let go, follow your lead, and completely submit to you. She doesn't have to think logically about anything because you're taking care of it all for her.

But it's important to give these commands in a confident way, without a seed of doubt in your mind. Their power lies in their confidence. If you give a weak command, she won't follow it.

Here are some commands you can use:

"Get on your knees and put my dick in your mouth." Sit on the edge of the bed or on a chair, and deliver this command.

"Get on top of me and ride this dick." Use this when you want her to get on top and ride you.

"Look at me while you suck it." Say this one while she's giving you head.

"Feel how hard you make me." I like to say this one to lead into sex. To do this, stand up next to the bed while she's sitting on the edge so that your dick is about face level with her. Then have her feel your erection from outside of your pants. Then, tell her to unbutton your pants, take it out, and suck it.

"Turn around and lie on your stomach." You can use this one when you want to move her into the doggy style position. I usually like to do this one simply by physically moving her, but you can also give this verbal command.

"Strip for me." There's nothing sexier than when a girl takes her clothes off slowly for you. She removes her shirt, then bends down in front of you as she takes her pants off. Use this when you want to see that beautiful sight. (Though I recommend using it when a girl is particularly sexy and confident in her body. Otherwise she may feel insecure about doing it.)

Experiment and make your own commands, too.

Remember that you can turn anything that you want to do in the bedroom into a command.

Pull Her Hair

Whenever you pull her hair, make sure to do it from the roots (i.e. the part closest to her head) rather than the ends of her hair. This makes it more pleasurable instead of painful and also avoids any potential neck injuries.

You should start light and notice how she responds to the hair pulling. If she likes it, then tug a little harder. If she doesn't (or if you realize she has extensions), then stop pulling her hair (not every girl likes it).

Here are some of the best times to pull her hair:

- **When you're fucking her doggy style,** pull her head back by her hair and kiss her neck.

- **When she's giving you head,** pull the roots of her hair as leverage for moving her back and forth on your dick.

- **When you're fucking her in *missionary with full contact*,** you can tug her hair back and lightly bite her neck.

Manhandle Her

Manhandling is a cornerstone of rough, dominant

sex.

It gives her just a little bit of pain while maximizing her psychological stimulation.

Just be sure that when you do it, you do it carefully, so you don't actually physically hurt her.

Here are some ways you can manhandle a woman during sex:

- Pick her up, have her wrap her legs around you, and pin her back against the wall while you fuck her.

- When she's riding you, put one arm around her waist and move her body up and down on your dick.

- Physically move her into different positions. For example, if you want to move from a bed position to fucking her against the wall, you can take her hand, walk over to the wall, pin her against it, and take her from behind.

Choke Her

This is one you have to be especially cautious with (for obvious reasons) but also one that a lot of women surprisingly love. Some women will even say, "Choke me!" during sex.

I recommend not trying this one out until you've had sex with a girl a few times (unless she blatantly tells you she wants it).

If and when you choke a girl, do so by putting pressure on the sides of her neck instead of her windpipe so you don't completely cut off her oxygen supply. Start gently, and be especially aware of her facial expressions to make sure she's okay, and don't choke her for more than twenty to thirty seconds at a time.

Spank Her

Of the hundreds of women I've been with, I'd say that roughly 90% (if not more) love to be spanked. In fact, I can't even remember a specific time when a girl didn't like it.

You can spank her when fucking her doggy style, while you're in the "69" position and her ass is near your face, and pretty much at any time during sex.

Start with a light spank, and if she likes it (or moans loudly), escalate a bit harder with each spank.

Bite Her

Biting can be very pleasurable for a girl...

You can bite her nipples, neck, shoulders, ears, and lips.

Start with soft bites, and if she reacts well, bite a little harder. Just try and avoid leaving a mark in an obvious place, like on her neck. And be careful when biting sensitives places like her nipples and lips.

Fuck Her Face

Somewhere along the line, I've learned a fact of life:

Some women like to get their face fucked.

They love it when you thrust into their mouth and literally fuck their face into submission. In fact, some of the most innocent-seeming girls I've met have been the ones who liked to get their face fucked the most.

Not sure if she likes to get her face fucked? Well, the better she is at giving head, the more likely she wants you to fuck her face.

Here's the best position to do it in:

Straddle her so that you're positioned right below her breasts. Lift her head up slightly and put your dick into her mouth. Then start thrusting lightly. If she responds well and seems to like it, go a bit harder.

Just be sure not to get too deep into her throat as this might cause her to throw up on your dick, and that's no fun.

Come on Her Face, in Her Mouth, and/or on Her Tits

I used to never do this.

"What if she doesn't want the cum on her face, mouth, or body?" I thought…

Then I dated a girl who literally begged me to come all over her face and body, and I thought, "This is fucking awesome. I need to do this more often."

There's something awesome about seeing a girl on her knees in front of you, mouth open and waiting to receive your load all over her. It's the ultimate show of dominance.

So now I do it probably 80-90% of the time. And the girls just about always oblige, get on their knees, and take the load. They'll do the same for you, too, if you're dominant enough.

However, until you get more experience with this, I recommend starting by coming on her tits.

Here's how to do it…

- When you realize you're about to finish, pull out and tell her you want to come all over her titties. It's better to say you want to come on her titties the first time you're having sex with a girl — that way you can gauge how down she is to get it on her face and in her mouth. If she's comfortable with your dick in the area of her face and titties when you're about to finish, then she's most likely cool with you finishing on her face. If she seems hesitant, then you can always come on her tits this time and go for the face the next time when you have more comfort built up with her.

- From here, you can either stand up and have her get on her knees (this is usually what I prefer), sit down on a chair or the edge of the bed and have her suck you off from there, or have her lie down on her back so you can fuck her face till you finish.

- Once you're on the very edge of coming, tell her you want to come all over her pretty face.

- Finish on her face, in her mouth, or on her tits, whichever you prefer.

Wrapping Up Dominance...

This is probably the most vulgar chapter so far in the book, and it may have even offended some people.

But you know what? Very few people are actually going to tell it to you like it is when it comes to sex and dominance. All the sexless virgins and ghostwriting chumps with pathetic Amazon books about sex – they are certainly not going to tell it to you this way because they wouldn't know good sex if it literally fucked them in the face.

I tell you about dominance based not on theory but on experience with hundreds of women. So, you can believe me or not, but for the guys who take this and put it to use, your sex life is going to transform, and you'll become the dominant man that the majority of women dream of. I can promise you that.

Anyway, I guess all this sex-writing has got me fired up. So I'll stop my tangent and give a quick recap of this chapter.

Here's the recap:

- Women don't like weak, vanilla men. They crave dominant men, and they want dominant sex.

- Just because a woman likes some dominant behavior (like getting her hair pulled and being spanked) doesn't mean she likes all dominant behavior. And just because she doesn't like one type of behavior doesn't mean she won't like any other types. Experiment and see what your girl likes most.

- In order to be dominant, you can do the following:

- Give her commands instead of asking for permission.

- Pull her hair from the roots.

- Manhandle her to give her a little bit of pain with maximized psychological pleasure.

- Choke her, but put pressure on the sides of her neck instead of her windpipe, and be very careful with this one.

- Spank her.

- Fuck her face by thrusting in and out of her mouth

(just make sure not to go too deep into her throat).

- Come on her face, in her mouth, and/or on her tits.

Okay, so dominance is clearly important. But you need more than dominance to give a girl a great sexual experience.

You need to balance it out with emotion. When you combine dominance and emotion, the sex goes from good to mind-blowing. And that's what we'll talk about next...

Fundamental #17: Emotion

Every woman has two sides...

A part that wants to be dominated, and a part that wants to experience a wide range of emotions.

If you're ALL dominance ALL the time, she won't be comfortable enough to fully give herself to you sexually.

She needs to feel passion, and for that, she needs an emotional connection.

That's a reason behind the popularity of romance novels. Women get wrapped up in the emotions of it all – they dream of a man who can induce the same types of emotions.

So, how do you give women that emotional experience in the bedroom? That's what this chapter is all about...

You'll learn how to give her an emotional and passionate experience in the bedroom. You can combine this with dominance and even switch back and forth between dominance and emotion to add variety to a sex session.

Let's dive in.

Connect with Her on an Emotional Level Before Sex

A lot of the emotional part of a sexual experience comes before you have sex. If you haven't connected with her on an emotional level beforehand, it'll be hard to do so during sex. You have no foundation to work from.

Here are some ways you can make that emotional connection before sex:

- **Talk about emotional topics that allow you to get to know her on a deeper level.** Topics like her experiences, her dreams, her passions, and what she loves to do.

- **Keep the conversation focused on her** so she feels invested in the interaction (because she doesn't usually reveal so much about herself).

- **Tease her occasionally** by doing things like accusing her of hitting on you and stereotyping her in a fun way (e.g. "Oh, you're a country girl? So what do you do when you're not square dancing?")

Look into Her Eyes

Eye contact is powerful, especially during sex.

You don't need to hold it the whole time, but

intermittent eye contact at the right moment will create an emotional experience.

For example, when fucking her in *missionary with full contact*, you can pull her head back and look into her eyes for ten to fifteen seconds.

French Kiss Her

When you share a French kiss during sex with a girl, it's a very intimate thing. Basically, what you're doing is giving her the sexual kiss we talked about before, except with a little more tongue.

Here are some great ways to start this kind of kiss during sex:

- Hold her hair tightly at its roots and kiss her in the *missionary with full contact* position.

- When fucking her doggy style, tug her hair back, turn her head sideways, and kiss her.

- When she's riding you on the edge of the bed while you're sitting up, draw her head towards yours and kiss her.

Moan and Grunt

I found this a bit surprising, but girls tell me over and over again that most guys are silent during sex. Maybe it's an ego thing, or maybe these guys just feel awkward. I'm not sure.

Here's what's interesting: just about every girl I've been with has loved that I moan during sex and oral sex. It pleasures them when they see that the experience (and what they're doing) is pleasuring me. Now, I'm not grunting like Venus and Serena Williams during a tennis match, but I'm doing enough to show that I'm very much enjoying the experience — and they love it.

Moaning, by the way, is a sound that you make when feeling pleasure. Grunting is a sound you make when exerting effort.

Here's how you can get started moaning and grunting if you've never done it before...

- Moan when she's giving you a blowjob.

- Moan when she's riding you.

- Grunt when you're fucking her really hard.

They key is to let it come out naturally. Don't force it. Allow it to be an expression of what you're feeling instead of a sound you're trying to manufacture in your head.

The more you do it, the more natural it will be.

Wrapping Up Emotion...

Emotion is an important part of a sexual experience with a girl. When you combine it with dominance, you can be a masterful lover.

Here's a recap of how to bring emotion into sex...

- Connect with her on an emotional level before sex. This will give you a foundation for making things more emotional and passionate during sex.

- Look into her eyes for ten to fifteen seconds while fucking her, and repeat this every couple of minutes.

- French kiss her to increase the level of intimacy.

- Moan and grunt to show her that you're enjoying the experience and that she's giving you pleasure.

Fundamental #18: The "Motion of the Ocean"

"There's something different about the way you fuck me," she said.

"Oh yeah? What's that?" I grinned.

"The way you move. The way our bodies sync up and seem to go in a perfect rhythm. It feels like we've been having sex for months even though we've only done it a few times," she replied.

"Girl, I wasn't joking when I said I have rhythm." I laughed.

***

You've probably heard of the saying, "It's not the size of the boat, it's the motion of the ocean."

Whoever came up with that saying understood the importance of good rhythm during sex.

Good rhythm makes the difference between an immersive sexual experience and an awkward, clunky combination of two people's genitals.

It's an absolute necessity for good sex. The problem is, a lot of guys don't quite have it. There's no flow to their sexual movements, and so the girl can never really get into it or have an orgasm.

But if you want to become a masterful lover, then you'll have to master your rhythm. And this chapter will show you how to do that.

Here's How You Can Develop More Rhythm...

First off, here are the elements that make up your rhythm during sex:

- The speed at which you thrust (fast vs. slow)

- The type of thrust (in and out vs. side to side vs. no thrust at all)

- The strength at which you thrust (hard vs. soft)

- How much you alternate between different types of thrusts (variety)

Keep these in mind as we get further into the rest of these tips for developing your rhythm.

Start with Slow Thrusts

Use slow thrusts at the beginning to set the pace and allow yourself to get into a good rhythm.

The slow thrusts help you ease into the sex and get a sense of her rhythm too. They also help you get more immersed in the experience. You can feel the full scope of the pleasure while maintaining control of the pace so you don't come too quickly.

Speed Up, Then Slow Back Down

As you get into a good flow with the slow thrusts after a minute or two, start to speed up. Go in and out with faster thrusts for a bit. This adds variety and intensity to the sex.

Then, slow back down after a bit.

You can alternate the speeds of your thrusts throughout the whole sex session. Just try to keep the thrusts steady. For example, don't do 3 quick thrusts, followed by 2 slow thrusts, followed by 2 more quick thrusts. Instead, for example, you can thrust quickly for a minute, slow down a bit for a minute, and then speed back up again. That way, you'll have enough time to get into a good rhythm at each speed.

Use the Music as a Guide

I play music almost every time I have sex, and I recommended you do the same (go back to the fundamental on transforming your apartment into a panty-dropping bachelor pad for a recap of this).

You can use the music as a guide for your thrusts.

You can speed up and slow down with the tempo. When you sync your bodies up with the music, it adds even more pleasure to the experience.

Use Your Hips

Ever heard the phrase, "It's all in the hips?" Well, when it comes to rhythm, the hips are one of your most important tools.

Use your hips to vary thrusts. Use them to thrust harder and to slow down, as well as to rotate while you're inside of her.

For a crash course on using your helps well, I recommend checking out some old Chris Brown dance videos. You know, the ones where he basically humps the floor. There's a reason this type of dancing drives women crazy.

Take a Latin Dance Class

I've gotten much better at sex in the last few years since living in Latin countries like Colombia and Mexico. And that's no coincidence.

I've learned to dance reggaeton, bachata, salsa, and more. With all of these Latin dances, you have to move your hips well and get the rhythm down.

This alone has taught me more about rhythm than any book or video ever could.

So I recommend taking a Latin dance class like salsa or bachata and hitting up a few Latin clubs that play reggaeton.

Dance with the girls there and experiment with the dance styles. In the process, you'll developna better sense of rhythm as well as some sexy dance moves. It's a win-win.

Wrapping Up the "Motion of the Ocean"...

Good rhythm, or as some call it, the "motion of the ocean", is essential to good sex.

Most guys don't have good rhythm, so simply by getting this down, you set yourself apart.

Here's a quick recap:

- Rhythm has to do with the speed, strength, and motion of your thrusts.

- Start with slow thrusts to set the pace and get into a good flow.

- Speed up your thrusts and then slow them back down to add variety and intensity to the sex.

- Use music as a guide and thrust to the tempo of the beat.

- Use your hips for more effective rhythmic thrusting.

- Take a Latin dance class like salsa, as this well help you develop a natural sense of rhythm.

Fundamental #19: Dirty Talk

Just as a steak isn't quite as tasty without the salt and pepper, sex isn't quite as good without a little spice.

And one of the most important spices to add into the mix is dirty talk. When used properly, it can enhance the sex for both you and your girl.

With it, you can turn up the dominance and emotion, both during foreplay and sex. You can also use it to give her multiple orgasms and increase the intensity of each of them.

But as with any spice, you have to use it in the right way and at the right moment. Otherwise, it can ruin the experience instead of enhancing it.

So, how do you use dirty talk the right way?

First, understand that dirty talk should not be logical, funny, or validation-seeking. These things will rip her out of the immersive experience and potentially turn her off.

For example, don't ask, "Do you like it?" Of course she likes it – there's no need to seek her validation. If you ask this, you'll seem insecure and unconfident in what you're doing.

The key is to say the right thing at the right time and to mean it. For example, when you're making out before sex, you can pull back, stare into her eyes, and say something like, "Babe, you're so beautiful." This will turn her on and further immerse her in the experience. But if you say the same thing while you're railing her from behind, and she's about to come, it's a little awkward.

It'd be a lot better to say something like, "You're my naughty little girl, and you're going to come all over me."

With this in mind, here are some ground rules for talking dirty in the bedroom:

- **Use possessive language.** This makes it more personal and intimate. For example, "You're my dirty little slut, aren't you?" is much better than, "You're a dirty slut," because it implies she only does those things with you.

- **Tell her what you want.** Tell her what you want her to do to you – it's that simple. For example, "Ride that dick like you mean it," or "Stand up and get against the wall."

- **Say it like you mean it.** You can't talk dirty in an insecure tone. You must speak with confidence and be sure of what you're saying. If she senses a hint of insecurity in your voice, it loses its power.

- **Tell her what you like.** This shows her what you like so she can do more of it and also pleases her by showing her that she's pleasing you. For example, you can say, "I love when you look up at me while you suck my dick," or, "Your ass drives me crazy."

- **Command her.** When you command her, she can let go, follow your lead, and completely submit to you. You can say things like, "Get on your knees and get ready to take my cum all over your face."

Keep in mind that dirty talk really depends on what you like and what you want to do during sex. It helps both you and the girl get more immersed in the experience. And so it's good to keep these ground rules in mind and just kind of make it up as you go and experiment with it. You'll learn to improve your dirty talk the more you do it.

But if you've never talked dirty before, you might find it difficult to get started. So, I'll give you some examples of dirty talk you can experiment with...

Foreplay Dirty Talk

- I'm going to fuck you until you can't walk.

- Get on your knees and take this dick in your mouth.

- Undress for me.

- Strip for me.

- Look up at me while you suck my dick.

- Spit on my dick.

- Use more hands.

- You're making me so hard right now.

- You taste so fucking good.

- Feel how hard you're making me.

Dirty Talk During Sex

- Ride me harder.

- Good girl (when she's doing something you like).

- You look so fucking sexy right now.

- Come for me, baby (when you see that she's close to coming).

- I can't wait to cum on your pretty little face.

- Tell me who owns this fucking pussy.

- Your tight little pussy drives me crazy.

- Bend over and show me that ass.

- Get on your hands and knees and get ready to take my dick.

Wrapping Up Dirty Talk...

Dirty talking helps you create a more immersive sexual experience. Done right, it makes the girl come more, come harder, and lose herself in the moment. It creates an intensity that is hard to reach with silent sex.

Here's a quick recap of the dirty talk fundamental:

- Use possessive language to make it more personal and intimate.

- Tell her what you want.

- Say it like you mean it – don't let uncertainty creep into your voice.

- Tell her what you like to show her that she's giving you pleasure.

- Command her so she can let go and follow your lead.

Fundamental #20: Variety

Variety is the spice of life, and as it turns out, it's also the spice of the bedroom.

It's important both within each individual sex session and over the course of all of your sex sessions in a relationship with a girl.

You shouldn't be doing the same things for the duration of every sex session. This will quickly get boring for both you and the girl you're having sex with. It'll just be so damn predictable. Nor should you do the same things over the course of multiple sex sessions in a relationship.

The same positions, the same time, the same location, etc. Eventually, sex will stop being fun.

But when you add variety, you can keep sex interesting and exciting, continue to have great sex even if you've been with a girl for a long time, and make sex more adventurous and enjoyable for yourself.

Luckily, it's quite easy to add variety, and there are plenty of ways to do it.

Here's how you can add more variety to sex:

Using Different Sex Positions

You've already got 10 different sex positions in your arsenal from this book, so you've got plenty to choose from and transition to.

And remember: you can use a position multiple times throughout the same session of sex.

You should switch positions every seven to ten minutes or so. This gives you enough time to enjoy the position and get into a good rhythm, but it's not so long that it starts to get boring. After seven to ten minutes, switch to another position and keep it going.

(For positions where you expend more energy, like if you fuck her while holding her up, you can go less than seven minutes. Otherwise, you might tire yourself out too quickly.)

Time of Day

What time of day do you usually have sex? For most people, it's later on in the evening.

There's no problem with that, but it's also good to switch it up once and while.

For example, if you usually have sex in the evening, have sex the next morning too. Or do it on your lunch break, or even in the middle of the night when you can't sleep.

When you switch up the time of day, sex becomes less predictable and a bit more exciting.

Duration

Switch up the amount of time you have sex for.

If you usually fuck your girl for thirty minutes to an hour, then you can surprise your girl with a five minute "quickie" before she goes into work.

Or you can go for two hours and have a marathon sex session.

Watching Porn

This is a great way to spice things up.

It helps to have a laptop, flat screen TV, and HDMI cable to make the experience more immersive.

Get naked, lie on the bed with your girl, and type in the URL of your favorite porn site. Spend some time watching and enjoying the porn together. The two of you can masturbate next to each other too.

Then, when you actually have sex soon after, you'll both be extremely turned on. You can leave the porn on in the background, as the background moans add a nice touch to the sexual experience with your girl.

Using Toys

Go to an erotica store with your girl and shop for sex toys.

Dildos, vibrators, cock rings, handcuffs, blindfolds, etc. There are plenty of tools you can use to spice things up.

For example, when fucking her doggy style, you can reach around and put the vibrator against her clit for extra stimulation.

You can also do things like handcuff her to the bed, watch her masturbate with a dildo, and even tie her down. Use your imagination!

Amount of Foreplay

You don't need to go through the full spectrum of foreplay before every sex session. In fact, sometimes it's good to skip it altogether and get right to the sex.

This will make your sex sessions less predictable, and it'll also make foreplay more enjoyable when you do it (because she won't be sure if it'll happen 100% of the time).

Amount of Skin-to-Skin Contact

Skin-to-skin contact increases intimacy, pleasure, and

passion during sex. But if you're always making skin-to-skin contact, then it'll become predictable, and the pleasure derived from it will fade.

So add variety here. The majority of the time, you can use positions with lots of skin-to-skin contact, but sometimes you can pull away and go for positions with less (or barely any) skin-to-skin contact.

Then, when you switch back from minimized skin contact to maximized contact, you'll enhance the pleasure derived from that contact.

Location

I stay in a different Airbnb apartment nearly every month, and the sex is always just a little bit more fun for the first time in that new apartment – especially if it's with a girl I'm dating.

There are new things to explore within it, like different mattresses, bean bags, tables, mirrors, etc.

The lesson? Location is one of the best ways you can add variety.

You can do it in different rooms within your apartment, do it in public, or even rent a hotel and do it there for a night.

Wrapping Up Adding Variety to Sex...

Variety is the spice of life, and it's key to a great sex life too.

It keeps sex interesting, unpredictable, and filled with different kinds of sensations.

You should have variety within individual sessions and also over the course of all your sex with a girl.

To recap, here are some ways you can add more variety to sex:

- Alternate between different sex positions every seven to ten minutes.

- Have sex for different amounts of time and at different times of day.

- Watch porn to amplify the mood before and during sex.

- Use sex toys like blindfolds, handcuffs, and vibrators.

- Use varying levels of foreplay.

- Use varying levels of skin-to-skin contact.

- Switch up locations between different apartments, rooms, and public places.

Fundamental #21: Orgasmic Anal Sex

I still remember my first anal sex experience…

I pulled a girl to my room from a frat party. I'd met her ten minutes beforehand and barely exchanged a few words with her. But it was clear what she wanted, and I was happy to oblige.

We started having sex on my couch, and she rode me for a few minutes. Then things took a surprising turn.

She got up, then got on her knees in front of the couch. She looked back and said, "I want it from behind" with a devious look. I thought, "Hmm… Is she talking about doggy style, or does she want it in the ass?"

I went with the safer option and started fucking her doggy style in her vagina. She turned around again and said, "No, I want you to fuck me in the ass."

In my drunken stupor, I thought, "Hmm. Not really an anal sex guy. Never done this before. Never really wanted to do it. But… fuck it. Adventure."

So I took it out of her vagina and started fucking her in the ass. It slipped right in with no problem, and she loved it. Hell, she even had multiple orgasms, which I didn't even know was possible from anal sex.

I later learned that anal sex isn't supposed to be this easy, and usually you need lube and preparation to do it right. But I guess this girl was a bit more... experienced in the anal sex department.

***

I've never been a big anal sex guy, but there's a time and a place for everything – and I know a lot of guys are really fascinated by the whole idea.

So I thought an anal sex fundamental would be a good addition to this book.

I've had some interesting anal sex adventures like the one above but also some with girls I really liked, where we discussed it and prepared beforehand. Usually the latter is better – there's more trust and comfort.

I'll lay out a few steps for having orgasmic anal sex...

Get Clean

Comfort is one of the biggest keys to anal sex. If she's not comfortable, she won't be able to open herself up and enjoy it, and this can lead to a painful experience.

And one of the best ways to make sure she's comfortable is to help her feel clean (even if she's already clean down there, which is probably the case). To do this, you can simply shower with her beforehand or have her use an anal douche.

Start Slow – Both Mentally and Physically

Bring up the topic beforehand and start getting her mentally prepared for it. Chances are, she's thought about having anal sex before, and she may have even had it in the past.

When bringing up the topic, you can discuss some of your past positive anal sex experiences and even watch some anal sex porn. This will help give her more positive feelings about it and make her more open to trying it with you.

Then, during foreplay, start playing with her anus and stick a finger in there. Gradually do this more and more so that she's more comfortable having you down there. That way, when it's time to have anal sex, she can loosen up easier.

When you start out the anal sex session, go slow as well. It can be painful at first, so slower thrusts are better, and they allow her to get used to having you inside her.

Have the Lube Ready

Don't go in there without any lube. Have some anal

lube ready and put it on her anus as well as on the condom before you start having sex.

This will make it much easier to penetrate her and take away from the initial pain she may feel when you put it in. Keep in mind that she doesn't naturally get wet down there like she does in her vagina.

Use the Right Positions

You'll need some different positions since you'll be going into her anus instead of her vagina.

Here are two of the best to go with (refer back to the sex position chapter to see how they look):

- The variation of the *scissor doggy style* position where both of her legs are together in the "savasana" position, and you're kneeling and penetrating her from behind.

- *Lying flat doggy style*

As you and your girl get more comfortable with anal sex, you can experiment with other positions like *reverse cowgirl, regular doggy style*, etc.

Thrust the Right Way

Tone down the dominant, hard thrusts when having anal sex. The act itself is dominant enough since it requires her to fully submit to you, and extremely hard thrusting can cause pain and bleeding.

Instead, use slower, rhythmic thrusts unless she tells you she wants it harder and faster. Even then, be careful so as not to hurt her.

How Does an Anal Orgasm Happen?

Yes, women can have orgasms from anal sex... but, how?

Well, remember the clitoris? It's a lot longer than you think. The part you see on the outside is just the tip – it actually extends further into her in a wishbone shape.

So when you have anal sex in the right positions, you actually stimulate her G spot and clitoris from behind. It's a little "back door" stimulation. And when you stimulate it enough through rhythmic thrusts, she can have an orgasm.

Wrapping Up Orgasmic Anal Sex...

Anal sex can be a good way to deepen the relationship between you and a girl, add variety to sex, and give both you and her a unique experience.

Here's a recap of orgasmic anal sex:

- Get cleaned up beforehand so she feels comfortable with you going down there.

- Start slow so she can be both mentally and physically prepared before you penetrate her.

- Have lube ready to make penetration easier and less painful.

- Use the right positions so that she can orgasm.

- Thrust with slow, rhythmic movements.

Part VI:
How to Last Longer, Stay Harder, and Beat Performance Anxiety

What It Takes to Last Longer (and the Roots of Performance Anxiety)

You now have a lot of tools in your arsenal for having mind-blowing sex.

But if you have debilitating performance anxiety, then all of those tools won't mean much. You won't be able to put them to good use!

We all get performance anxiety from time to time. As you get more sexual experience, however, performance anxiety becomes rarer and rarer.

But you need to know how to beat performance anxiety whenever it pops up.

The whole reason for it is that you're too in your head. It's a mental thing.

You're focusing on thoughts instead of being present in the moment.

"What if I finish too early? What's she going to think of me? This is going to be so embarrassing!"

These thoughts rob you of the experience of great sex.

This part of the book will show you how to beat performance anxiety so you can consistently have great sex.

But first, you should understand the roots of performance anxiety...

The Roots of Performance Anxiety

Depending on the guy, performance anxiety can be narrowed down to one or more of the following:

- Insecurity about penis size.

- Insecurity about how long you can last.

- Insecurity about getting a boner.

- Insecurity about lack of sexual experience.

First, a note on penis size...

 When it comes to penis size, many men are insecure that they're not big enough, and their "tool" won't be able to please a woman. This makes sense, because guys have been programmed by porn to believe that women only like abnormally large penises.

Most women I talk to, however, tell me they prefer a more average-sized penis. It fits better, is more versatile, and they can do more without it being painful.

So if you have an average or even below average tool, don't beat yourself up about it. You can easily make up for the lack of size with good rhythm, dominance, and all the other fundamentals we talked about earlier.

And one more note on insecurity about how long you last…

It's not so much that you need to last a specific amount of time. There is no specific "perfect duration" for sex. It's more about being able to control your orgasm so you can last as long (or as short) as you want.

You're going to learn how to do that in this part as well as how to beat the other insecurities I mentioned, too.

So let's get into the performance fundamentals!

Fundamental #22: Good Stamina and Breath Control

Like I said at the beginning of this book, you don't need to last for hours to have great sex. But you do need to last for more than a few minutes.

A five minute quickie is fun every now and then – and can even make for a good surprise for your woman (as I talked about earlier in the part about variety). But if you do that every time, it'll become a problem. You won't be able to deliver the kind of sex your woman craves, and she'll eventually look elsewhere for that sexual satisfaction.

Lasting longer in bed is something I had trouble with for a while. I'd go on streaks where I had no problem lasting as long as I wanted, followed by streaks where I could barely last 10 minutes.

But over time, as I slept with more girls, became more in tune with myself, and learned more about great sex, this stopped being a problem. Now, I can just about always last as long as I want. And I can tell you this: sex is A LOT more enjoyable when you have good stamina, and you're not worried about finishing too early all of the time.

So, how do you improve your stamina and last longer in bed? Here are some tips:

Be in the Moment

When you worry yourself about finishing too quickly, you're probably going to finish too quickly. Thoughts will swirl in your head like, "This is going to be so embarrassing" or, "She's going to judge me."

Instead, allow yourself to enjoy the sensations of sex and be in the moment. One thing that helped me a TON with this was meditation because, when you meditate, you practice being in the moment. After meditating for 10 minutes a day with Headspace for a month or two, my orgasm control dramatically improved.

Control Your Breathing

When you lose control of your breath, you're bound to lose control of your orgasm soon after. Meditation can help you control your breath as well. Another thing that can help is to actually count your breaths up to ten (and then repeat a few times) while you're having sex.

This makes you present with your breath. It's much easier to control it when you're actively aware of it.

Switch Positions

There are some sex positions that will just make you lose control, while others will get you exhausted. If you feel yourself starting to lose control too early, switch up the position to one with a little less stimulation or one that requires less physical exertion.

You can also pull out for a minute and go down on the girl. This allows you to accomplish two things: One, you give her clit some extra stimulation, and two, you help yourself to sexually "recharge" and seize back control of your orgasm.

Don't Thrust All the Time

You don't have to thrust constantly. Sometimes you can slow it down and, instead of thrusting, move in a circular motion for twenty to thirty seconds. This provides good stimulation for the girl while lessening your own stimulation (because you're not thrusting in and out).

You can also stop moving altogether and hold yourself inside of her a little deeper for thirty seconds or so (if you're on the bigger side, just make sure not to go too deep as this can be very painful for the girl). While doing this, you can kiss her neck and breasts.

Stop Cycling Through Sexual Techniques in Your Head

This will take you out of the present moment. Instead, internalize these fundamentals.

In other words, you won't have to be thinking, "Okay I did X, now it's time to try this other technique." Instead, you'll just need to think, "Okay, more dominance. Okay, now more variety. Etc." until it becomes completely natural.

Hit the Gym Consistently

You should be lifting weights and doing a little cardio. This will improve your actual stamina so that you have the energy to fuck a girl for thirty minutes to an hour.

I'm not a big fan of running, whether it be going for a jog or running on the treadmill. Either way, it sucks for me. I prefer to get my cardio through sports. And so I make it a point to play pickup basketball two to three times a week.

(Keep in mind I manage to do this while living in three to four countries every year. There are recreational pickup sports in just about any big city — you just need to ask around and/or do a little searching online. For example, a quick search for Budapest basketball led me to the "Budapest Basketball International" Facebook group. I now play with these guys every week while I'm in Hungary.)

Wrapping Up Good Stamina and Breath Control...

You don't need to last for hours to have great sex, but you don't want to be a "minute man" either.

Use these tips to build your sexual stamina so you can last for as long as you want to.

To recap:

- Be in the moment so you can enjoy the experience without psyching yourself out.

- Control your breathing so you can pace yourself and avoid exhaustion.

- Switch to a less stimulating position if you feel like you're losing control, and switch to a less physically exerting position if you feel like you're getting tired too quickly.

- Don't thrust constantly – slow down, rotate, and use other movements.

- Don't cycle through sexual techniques in your head.

- Hit the gym a few times a week to improve your physical stamina.

Fundamental #23: Get a "Main Girl"

Lack of sexual experience is one of the big insecurities that leads to performance anxiety.

If you haven't had a lot of sex, it's difficult to be confident that you can do it well (no matter how many books you read on the subject).

But this problem can be easily solved. How?

By getting a "main girl."

Your main girl doesn't have to be your girlfriend. She can just be a girl that you have sex with somewhat regularly (i.e. one or more times per week).

This will help you to gain sexual confidence and get more sexual experience. You'll learn what she likes in the bedroom, and you'll also learn more about what you like.

Your main girl basically provides a comfortable sexual environment for you to gradually improve in.

As you apply the fundamentals you've already learned with her, you'll get more comfortable having sex, get better at it, and naturally start to last longer and give her more orgasms.

I had a main girl when I lost my virginity and have had several main girls since then. Very few of them had the "girlfriend" label, but we had sex regularly. When I look at the periods of my life when I made the biggest strides in terms of getting better at sex, it's almost always the periods when I had a main girl.

Now, you might be wondering, "How do I get a main girl?"

If so, take another look at the first few parts of this book. They will help you become a more sexual man who attracts women with ease.

You can also check out any of the hundreds of articles on my blog, **PostGradCasanova.com**, and discover how to talk to women, date more women, start conversations, and a lot more.

Fundamental #24: Practice Vulnerability

A lot of men take themselves a little too seriously in the bedroom.

I know I used to do this. Maybe you can relate…

Guys feel like if they come too early or can't get a boner, then it's the end of the world.

Here's the thing: No matter how much you perfect your sexual abilities, you'll have situations where you'll come before you want to or when you can't get it up.

It happens to all of us.

And the worse you react to this – the more you make it seem like a big deal – the worse you'll make the situation.

For example, if you come too quickly and keep saying, "I can't believe this! This never happens. I usually last as long as I want. Trust me, I'm a lot better than this," the girl is going to feel like it probably *does* happen all the time.

The same goes for if you can't get a boner and react similarly.

It's far better to practice vulnerability instead.

Here's what I mean by that...

Instead of resisting the fact that it happened, just accept it.

Stay calm and composed, and be honest with the girl.

For example, if you come too early, you can say "Ah, I lost control there. The way you rode me with your tight little pussy drove me crazy. I guess we'll have to go for round two in a little while" and give her a sly smile.

If you can't get it up, you can say "I guess I'm just a little nervous/tired/drunk right now. Let's chill out and try again in a little while (or in the morning)."

The biggest thing is to keep a calm, sort of nonchalant attitude about it. If you don't make it a big deal, then she won't make a big deal. And when you try again later on, you can fuck her better.

Fundamental #25: Get Harder Erections

There's nothing that kills a sex session faster than a flaccid penis.

On the flip side, an extra hard erection allows you to fuck her harder, deeper, and with more intensity.

But a lot of guys have trouble getting extremely hard erections. They get hard enough to have sex, but because they're not 100% hard, the sex isn't nearly as good.

Maybe you've had trouble getting erections in the past, or perhaps you just don't get quite as hard as you'd like (at least, not consistently).

If that's the case, you might be victim to some of these "erection killers":

- **Stress.** When you're anxious from day-to-day things, it's difficult to get in the moment. Then you start getting stressed about your erection difficulties, and it becomes a vicious cycle.

- **Lack of sleep.** A 2009 study of 401 men with sleep apnea found that 70% of those men had erectile dysfunction, which led researchers to believe that lack of sleep and erectile dysfunction are connected

[1]. When you're tired and groggy, you don't have the energy you need to perform well in bed, and you may not even be able to get it up.

- **Performance anxiety.** When you've got performance anxiety, you're in your head afraid that you won't perform well. This doesn't allow you to immerse yourself in the moment, and it can be so intense that it kills your ability to get hard.

- **Low testosterone.** Testosterone plays a big factor in a man's sex drive and performance. It's not the only factor, and you can still get a hard erection with low testosterone. However, low testosterone can affect your libido and sap your sex drive. So getting your testosterone levels in line can be helpful for getting harder erections.

- **Masturbating too much/overuse of porn**. When you masturbate daily or even multiple times a day to internet porn, you desensitize yourself to physical intimacy. A study by the Italian Society of Andrology and Sexual Medicine found that overuse of porn can lead to a drop in libido and make it difficult to get erections [2].

- **Alcohol/drugs.** That whole "whiskey dick" thing isn't a myth. According to a study by Brown University, alcohol directly affects the penis by interfering with parts of the nervous system that are essential for arousal and orgasm [3].

Even if you haven't had issues with getting erections, chances are you will at some point, especially as you get older. And you'll have to deal with the very issues I just pointed out.

So, here are some things you can do to combat these and get harder erections...

Go to the Gym

Not only will going to the gym make you look better and improve your physique (so you naturally attract more women), it will also increase testosterone and help you stay at a proper weight.

Both of these things aid in giving you harder erections.

You don't need to be a gym rat or a meat head. Simply aim to go to the gym two to three times a week and get a consistent lifting routine.

There are plenty of routines you can find online, but I recommend this routine from my friend David de las Morenas of How to Beast: **https://www.howtobeast.com/get-jacked/**

I lived with David for a year, and he helped me completely transform my physique with a program very similar to this one. And now I have more energy, a better physique, and more confidence in my physical appearance.

Get Better Quality Sleep

Sleep is key to your health and essential to your ability to get harder erections.

Most guys don't get enough sleep, and the quality of sleep they do get is quite low. So it's no surprise that when it comes time to get a hard erection, they don't perform consistently.

But there are a few simple things you can do to immediately start getting more quality sleep:

- **Sleep in a blacked out room.** Get blackout curtains (or a quality sleep mask) and put dark tape over little lights in your room (like a digital clock light).

- **Keep your bed time consistent.** This is easier said than done, especially if you like to go out on the weekends. But at the very least, try and go to bed at the same time every night during the week, ideally at a time that allows you to get in a solid eight hours of sleep.

- **Wear blue light blocking glasses before bed.** A recent study from Harvard University showed that blue light (i.e. the type of light that gets emitted from your phone and laptop) negatively affects your circadian rhythm, which can damage your sleep pattern [4]. So either avoid looking at digital screens for an hour before bed, or get a pair of blue light blocking glasses to mitigate their effects. I personally wear these blue light blocking glasses most nights before I go to bed: **http://amzn.to/2vTgvWV**

- **Avoid late-night meals.** It's tempting to hit that 24-hour McDonald's on your way home – trust me, I've been there before. While that late-night meal is satisfying in the moment, it can cause your blood sugar to spike, which interferes with your ability to get deep, quality sleep. So, it's best to fight those cravings and avoid late-night meals.

- **Have a "pre-sleep" routine**. Just as a good morning routine can help you crush the day, a good pre-sleep routine can help prepare you for quality sleep. Here are some habits you can put into that routine: reading, meditation, writing in a journal, and unplugging from TV/the phone.

Avoid Processed Foods and Refined Sugars

You probably have a sense of the foods that make you feel good and the foods that sap you of energy.

For example, you can feel the difference in your energy levels after you eat a healthy meal filled with whole foods (like grass-fed meat and veggies), versus a meal like pizza and soda.

I'm not a diet expert, but I've noticed that as I've improved my diet and cut out processed foods and refined sugars, I get harder erections and have much higher energy levels.

In general, you'll probably feel better if you stick to a diet filled with more whole foods than processed foods. So aim for things like grass-fed beef, wild-caught fish, and organic vegetables. Foods like these will give you energy (instead of sap it).

Drink Responsibly (or Not at All)

Every time I go out, I see dudes getting absolutely obliterated with alcohol. They drink until they can barely stand up anymore.

This leaves me scratching my head because they basically ruin their ability to be socially sharp, and if they somehow bring a girl home, they probably won't be able to get an erection.

Instead of drinking a ton when you go out, mix in some soda waters to stay hydrated and slow down your drinking pace. Hell, you can cut out the drinking altogether, save yourself money, and give yourself the health benefits of avoiding alcohol.

But at the very least, aim to keep it down to 1-4 drinks so that you keep a manageable buzz going but don't go over your limit. That way, you'll stay socially sharp and can get hard if you end up bringing a girl home.

Cut Down On the Porn/Masturbation

Masturbation – we all do it from time to time. Some of us more than others.

It can seem like a harmless thing – what's a little porn going to do, anyway? But as I mentioned earlier, it gradually desensitizes you to physical intimacy.

I'm not saying you need to cut it out completely, but try to limit it to 1-3 times a week or even less. At some point, you should be getting sex consistently enough to where you don't even think of looking at porn.

Wrapping Up How to Get Harder Erections...

When you can get harder erections, you can fuck your woman harder, stronger, and better. You'll avoid the disappointment that a flaccid penis brings and perform consistently at your best.

Here's a recap of how to get harder erections:

- Understand the factors that kill erections, like lack of sleep, low testosterone, stress, performance anxiety, and overuse of porn.

- Go to the gym to improve your physique and boost your testosterone.

- Get better quality sleep so you have high energy throughout the day and night.

- Avoid shitty foods that weigh you down and sap your energy.

- Drink less (or not at all) so that you're socially sharper and can perform well if you bring a girl home.

- Cut down on the porn/masturbation so that you don't desensitize yourself to physical intimacy.

Reference:

1. Budweiser, S., Enderlein, S., Jörres, R. A., Hitzl, A. P., Wieland, W. F., Pfeifer, M., & Arzt, M. (2009, November). Sleep apnea is an independent correlate of erectile and sexual dysfunction. From https://www.ncbi.nlm.nih.gov/pubmed/19570042

2. Scientists from the Italian Society of Andrology and Sexual Medicine: Too Much Internet Porn May Cause Impotence. (n.d.). from **http://www.foxnews.com/health/2011/02/25/scie ntists-internet-porn-cause-impotence.html**

3. Borreli, L. (2015, October 15). Alcohol And Sex: What Is 'Whiskey Penis' And How Does It Affect The Male Libido? From http://www.medicaldaily.com/alcohol-and-sex-what-whiskey-penis-and-how-does-it-affect-male-libido-357278

4. Blue light has a dark side. (n.d.). Retrieved October 30, 2017, from https://www.health.harvard.edu/staying-healthy/blue-light-has-a-dark-side

Fundamental #26: Use These Tips to Last Longer

A lot of what you've already learned in this book — from the sexual mindsets to stamina control, to practicing vulnerability — is going to help you last longer in bed.

But I wanted to lay out some concrete tips and put them in one place so you can go back to it whenever you're having a "lasting long" issue.

So keep these tips in mind — they'll come in handy whenever you feel like you're going to finish too soon.

Let's dive in...

Use Less Sensitive Positions

There are certain positions that make it harder to control yourself than others. These positions can vary from girl to girl and from session to session.

For example, some girls know how to ride a dick incredibly well. They work your tool like a joystick, effortlessly moving back and forth and maximizing pleasure for the both of you. But the catch is, these girls can go a little too fast and make you lose control. If you feel this happening, you can sit up some, grab her ass, and try to slow her movements down for a little bit.

Other girls, however, are tamer when they're on top, which makes it easier for you to last longer. Like I said, it depends on the girl.

And if the girl has a particularly nice ass, then doggy style might be the position that makes you lose control. Just be aware and be ready to change it up (or slow it down) before you feel like you're going to lose control.

Immerse Yourself

One of the biggest reasons why you come quickly is because you're thinking about NOT coming quickly. Instead, focus on your pleasure and being in the present moment with your girl.

Orgasm happens at some point in the future, but you're not thinking about the future. You're feeling everything in this moment. You are immersed.

When you immerse yourself, everything becomes easier. And it's a lot more pleasurable than trying to think about baseball!

Stop and Relax

This one is simple. When you feel like you're getting

close to finishing, stop thrusting. Relax, and allow her to feel you deep inside for a moment until your urge to come has completely subsided.

You can also pull out and eat her pussy for a minute or two – this will also give you time to calm down and recharge.

Go Multiple Rounds

Lost control and came too quickly the first time around? Calm down – it's not a big deal.

Give yourself fifteen to twenty minutes (or however long you need) to recharge. After you've already come once, it becomes easier to control your orgasm the second time around.

Use "Long-Lasting" Condoms (as a Last Resort)

Save this one as a last resort in case nothing else works. I say that because long-lasting condoms can take a little too much pleasure out of the sexual experience.

They use numbing lubricant, which basically numbs your penis so you can't feel as much. It can help you last longer, but it won't feel nearly as good.

Wrapping Up Tips to Help You Last Longer...

The more comfortable you get with sex, the easier it will be to last longer. And if you practice the fundamentals in this book, you'll eventually be able to last as long as you want just about every time you have sex.

That thought of "What if I come too early?" will pretty much never cross your mind again. And if by chance you do come too quickly (which happens to all of us from time to time), you can always relax a little bit and go for another round once you've recharged!

Here's a quick recap of the "last longer" tips:

- Use less sensitive positons when you feel like you're about to come so that you can regain control before it's too late.

- Immerse yourself in the sexual experience and be in the moment instead of constantly thinking about when you're going to come

- Stop and relax if you feel like the urge to come is getting overwhelming.

- Go multiple rounds. That way, if you come too quickly the first time, you can make it up to the girl in the next round.

- Use long-lasting condoms as a last resort – be careful, though, as they have numbing lubricants that dull pleasure and make sex a little less fun.

262

Part VII: What to Do After Sex

Fundamental #27: Show Her You Care

You now have all the tools you need to become amazing at sex.

Once you put these fundamentals into action, you'll give women mind-blowing orgasms and achieve the type of sexual lifestyle I described at the beginning of this book.

But before you go out and apply all of these things, I want to leave you with one final note…

The better you get at sex, the more women will feel connected to you, and the more they'll want to be with you.

Why? Well, think about it…

Women have all these disgustingly mediocre men hitting them up every day and on every medium (Facebook, texting, Instagram, and more). Just ask any girl and she'll show you the conversations. These mediocre men seek only validation and the chance to take advantage of the women they fawn after.

Women are tired of these pathetic men and even more tired of the pathetic advances they try to make. And on the occasions when a girl gives in to a mediocre man's advances, she's left unsatisfied after a night of mediocre sex.

It's rare that a woman meets a man who genuinely cares and is a masterful lover. It's a breath of excellence amidst a sea of mediocrity.

She recognizes this and has more admiration for this type of man. She opens herself up more, is vulnerable, and desires to connect more and more deeply with this kind of man.

You are on your way to becoming this man.

That's why it's important to treat her well after sex – both in the immediate aftermath as you lie next to her and in the days following.

Why? Well, it benefits both you and her.

By treating her well, you make her feel good about having been with you. Instead of regret and sexual shame (which some guys surely make her feel by acting the way they do), she'll feel a rush of good emotions, and she'll look back on it as a positive experience.

You'll show her that a guy can be great at sex and also genuinely care about her well-being. This will benefit her future relationships and honestly just make the world a bit of a better place.

And treating her well benefits you because it

improves your chances of seeing her again (if that's what you want), builds your reputation (she'll say good things about you to her friends), and doesn't give you the slimy feeling of manipulating a girl (in other words, it provides you with positive emotions, too).

It also makes it more likely that she'll feel comfortable chasing after you for more sex and desire to please you more and more.

So in this chapter, I'll show you the right way to treat a girl after sex. You'll learn the mistakes that a lot of guys make, and then I'll show you how to show her you care.

Let's get into it...

Common Mistakes Guys Make After Sex

They Make Her Feel like a Slut

Guys do this both intentionally and unintentionally. Chances are, you have done it unintentionally in the past.

Here are some things guys do to make her feel like a slut after sex:

- Say "thank you" like the girl just provided some sort of service for them.

- Ask her to leave right away.

- Say things like, "I can't believe you had sex with me so quickly."

- Ask questions like, "Do you usually sleep with guys on the first night?"

- Turn over and go to sleep immediately.

They Get Up and Leave Immediately

It's the old "fuck n' run" tactic. Right after you finish, you say, "Ah, I gotta go, but this was fun," and bolt out the door. This makes her feel like she just got used for sex.

They Bring Up Weird Conversation

They ask weird questions, make uncomfortable comments, and overall just act differently than they did before the sex.

How to Show Her You Care

Now that you know the common mistakes to avoid, let's talk about some things you can do to show her you care...

Help Her Clean Up

When the sex is over, things can be pretty messy — especially if you finish on her face and/or chest.

Have a roll of paper towels nearby, grab one, and wipe it off of her so she doesn't have to sit there covered in cum.

If You Ask Her to Leave, Do so Nicely

Let's be honest – there are times when you want to sleep alone, and you just don't want the girl to stay over much longer. That's fine – it's human.

In that case, you can ask her to leave, just don't be a dick about it.

I suggest lying there with her for five to ten minutes, then telling her you had a great time, but you want to get some sleep. Offer to walk her out and call her an Uber.

Tell Her She Can Stay If She Wants To

If you genuinely enjoyed your experience with her and don't mind if she sticks around, then tell her she can stay if she wants to. This is a great way to show her you care, especially if it's late at night and her only other option is to take a long taxi ride home.

Go for Another Round

When you go for round two, it tells her that you genuinely enjoyed the first round of sex. Your desire for her didn't diminish just because you'd already "gotten the notch in your belt."

Go for Breakfast the Next Day

This is one of the best ways to solidify a second meeting with a girl – especially if you just met her the night before, and she only knows you in a nightlife type of situation.

It gives you the chance to make it real with her and have some relaxed conversation. As a result, she's a lot less likely to feel like a slut afterwards.

Send Her a Follow-Up Text the Next Day

As a general rule, you should text girls the day after you have sex. This meshes with what I've been saying throughout this chapter – it shows that you're not just using her for the sex and that you actually care about her well-being.

You can say something as simple as, "Hey Ana, I had fun hanging out last night!"

Wrapping Up Showing Her You Care...

It's really not too difficult to show a girl that you care, and it benefits both you and the girl.

Here's a quick recap of this fundamental:

- When you treat her well, it gives the girl positive emotions, improves your chances of seeing her again, and increases her desire to please you.

- Avoid the common mistakes that most guys make, like asking her to leave immediately, acting weird, and asking weird questions.

- Show her you care by doing things like helping her clean up after sex, going for another round, and sending her a follow-up text the next day.

The Hook Up Handbook

Fundamental #28: Ask Her the Right Questions After Sex

The moments after sex are an interesting time. You're both clouded with feel-good endorphins, and she's probably feeling some more intense emotions than usual.

In this feel-good state, she's more likely to reveal stuff she may not normally talk about (especially if the sex was good). Specifically, things that can give you a clearer picture of who she is and what she likes in bed, as well as things that tell you what you did right during your interaction with her (so you can keep learning and improving your ability with women).

But she's usually not going to just reveal that stuff out of the blue. You have to ask her the right questions.

So in this chapter, I'll give you a few questions to consider asking while you lay next to her after the first sex session.

Don't hammer out these questions back-to-back like an interview. Ask one and let the conversation flow –

it'll eventually lead you into the other questions (and you certainly don't have to ask them all after the first session).

And keep in mind that her answers will help you to provide an even better sexual experience for her the next time around.

So, here are some questions to consider asking a girl after sex…

1. What's Your Favorite Sex Position?

This tells you what positions to focus more on the next time around. You can even dive deeper and ask about her favorite position for coming.

You may be surprised to learn that girls vary greatly in terms of their favorite positions. Some love to get fucked doggy style, while others love to come when they're riding you. So, it's good information to know for the next round of sex. You might even learn a new position from her.

2. What's a Sexual Fantasy You've Always Had?

Every girl has sexual fantasies. A girl's fantasies tell you about the type of sex she likes, what turns her on, and what kind of sexual experiences she may be open to.

And occasionally, depending on the fantasy, you may even be able to help her fulfill it.

If and when she tells you her fantasies, though, make sure not to appear judgmental at all. It's important to show her that you're open and that you don't judge women for their sexual desires. That way, she'll be comfortable experiencing and sharing more, and potentially even helping you fulfill your own sexual desires.

3. How Rough Do You Like It (i.e. hair pulling, choking, spanking, etc.)?

Most girls like rough sex at least a little bit. While you may not go as rough as you usually do during the first session, you can use this question to get a sense of how rough she wants it the next time around.

Again, you'll see a lot of variation with this. For example, some girls love to get their hair pulled, while others loved to get spanked and choked.

When you ask the question, you can act it out a bit too to make it more clear. For example, if she asks, "What do you mean by rough?", you can grab her by the root of her hair and say, "Like getting your hair pulled," then grab her ass and say, "or getting spanked."

4. At What Point Did You Realize You Wanted to Have Sex with Me?

This question is more meant for you. Usually girls will tell you they don't know the specific point – it just sort of happened.

But occasionally you'll get an answer like, "When you gave me that sexy stare in the bar, it really turned me on," or "You grabbed the root of my hair when you kissed me and I knew right then." These are the kinds of things that will give you insight into what you're doing well (and what you should do more of in the future).

5. Where's the craziest place you've ever had sex?

This one will give you insight into just how sexually open she is. It can also give you some ideas for sex in kinkier types of places, like on the beach, in a car, in public, etc.

You can use these ideas to spice up your sex life and add variety to your sessions with her.

6. How many people have you had sex with?

Note: This is one you should be cautious with.

Whether you ask it or not really depends on how much you care about her sexual history. If it's a big factor for you, then this is probably the best time to ask it, primarily because it's your best chance to get an honest answer.

The longer you hang out with a girl and they more she starts to like you, the more risk she'll feel about revealing her true sexual history (especially if she's been with her fair share of men). But after the first sex session, she's feeling those good endorphins and she's feeling open. It doesn't feel like a huge risk for her to reveal some of her sexual history because she isn't all that invested in you yet – she's only had sex with you one time.

As for whether or not you should care about her sexual history, that's a whole other topic and it depends on your preference.

And one more note: her version of the "truth" of her answer may be different than the actual truth. She might not count the random guy from that Mexico vacation, nor the college hook up where the guy put "just the tip" in.

7. Have you ever hooked up with a woman?

Whether you ask this question or not depends on whether you're open to the idea of a threesome with this girl and potentially another girl.

A surprising amount of girls have hooked up with other girls, or at least are open to doing it in the future. Still, others haven't done it and aren't open to it. This question gives you a good gauge on whether or not a threesome could be on the table at some point.

Wrapping Up Questions You Can Ask Her After Sex...

Right after a session of great sex, you're both feeling

good emotions and you're more open to each other. It's a golden opportunity to discover more about her sexual preferences, history, fantasies, and more.

To recap the questions you can ask her after sex:

1. What's your favorite sex position?

2. What's a sexual fantasy you've always had?

3. How rough do you like it?

4. At what point did you realize you wanted to have sex with me?

5. Where's the craziest place you've ever had sex?

6. How many people have you had sex with?

7. Have you ever hooked up with a woman?

Epilogue:
A Sunrise over
Medellin

We sat in bed, gazing out the window at the beautiful skyline of Medellin, Colombia. Ana and I had spent the last 3 months together adventuring around the country, having incredible sex, and sharing an amazing connection.

She was an innocent-looking, cute, and petite Mexican girl with short black hair and big natural breasts.

This was our last morning together. She had to fly back to Mexico later that day, and I was set to fly off to the United States soon after. We knew we'd probably never see each other again.

"What am I going to do?" she asked.

"What do you mean?" I said.

"What am I going to do if I never see you again and never get to have sex with you again? You're the best sex I've ever had… I don't think other guys are going to be able to do it like you…" she mused.

I thought back to the many girls with whom I'd had

mediocre sex. The times where I'd laid in bed, disappointed and slightly embarrassed for a lackluster performance.

Then I looked back over at her. She lay there in a state of complete satisfaction.

There's something awesome about lying next to a beautiful girl after a long night of amazing sex. As you both pant and regain your breath, you know you've given each other what you needed in that moment.

You know that you've ravished her the way a man is supposed to ravish a woman. You've provided her with an experience that all the mediocre men out there can only dream of – and one that she won't soon forget.

I shot Ana a devilish grin.

"Yeah, maybe you're right. Or hell, maybe one day, I'll write a book about it…"

A Final Recap

Fundamental #1: The Surface Level of Your Sexy Vibe

- Talk slower so you appear more confident and women hang on your words.

- Move slower to come across as more sexually appealing and controlled.

- Pause at the right time to build tension.

- Master the sexy smile instead of cheesing like Urkel.

- Deepen your tone of voice by speaking from your belly.

Fundamental #2: The Physical Level of Your Sexy Vibe

- Work on your physique so you look better and have more sexual stamina.

- Develop your style and wear clothes that fit well.

- Get a good haircut to be more physically appealing, and keep your facial hair well-groomed.

Fundamental #3: The Deeper Level of Your Sexy Vibe

- Develop your charisma so that you come off as more interesting, intriguing, and sexy.

- Develop an authentic sense of humor so that you look at life positively and have a good attitude.

- Become more independent and stop relying on other people for your own happiness.

- Live a purposeful life so that you have greater aspirations than simply being with a woman.

Fundamental #4: The Sexual Mindsets

- "I can enjsoy a woman's presence without the need for sex."

- "I won't always perform at my best, and that's okay."

- "I can give women an amazing sexual experience."

Fundamental #5: Escalate Through "Sexy Talk"

- Use sexual humor – but remember to be subtle and throw in the occasional innuendo.

- Speak with intent to convey your sexual vibe and turn her on.

- Look at her lips to get her thinking about sex.

- Connect on a deeper level to earn her trust and make the sex better later on.

Fundamental #6: Recognize When She's Horny (and Wants You to Make a Move)

- She's receptive to your touch and touches you back.

- She gets in your personal space (and is comfortable with you in hers).

- She talks less and gives shorter answers.

 - The two of you are alone in private.

- She holds lingering eye contact.

Fundamental #7: Turn Her On from the First Kiss

- Go in for the kiss the right way, and pull away after a few seconds.

- Master the sexual kiss so you can turn her on and get her thinking of sex.

Fundamental #8: Transform Your Apartment into a Panty-Dropping Bachelor Pad

- Keep your apartment clean.

- Cultivate a good ambiance by using warm lighting and chill music.

- Have the right-sized bed equipped with comfortable bedding.

- Make sure you've got condoms and lube ready.

Fundamental #9: Know Her Most Important Parts

- The clitoris is filled with nerve endings and gets firmer and larger as the girl gets more stimulated.

- The labia minora and labia majora are the inner and outer lips of the labia.

- The G spot is a small patch of flesh located around two to three inches up inside the vagina on the front of the vaginal wall.

Fundamental #10: Master the Art of the Sexual Massage

- Get the right tools, like scented candles, incense, massage oil, and good music.

- Start the massage with her middle to upper back, shoulders, arms, and hands.

- Make the massage sexual by stroking her legs and turning away from her pussy at the last moment.

Fundamental #11: The "Finger Dance" That Makes Her Squirt

- Keep the ground rules in mind, like having well-groomed hands, teasing her beforehand, and starting slow.

- The more comfortable a girl is with you, the easier it will be for her to squirt.

- The "finger dance" and the slider are two great techniques to keep in mind when fingering a girl.

- Experiment yourself to see what each girl likes best.

- Some girls like anal play, so keep that in mind if you're into that kind of thing, too.

Fundamental #12: The Casanova Guide to Cunnilingus

- Tease her before the cunnilingus by kissing her erogenous zones, giving her a sexual massage, using your fingers, and kissing around her vagina.

- Keep the cunnilingus basics in mind, like starting slow, hitting the clit from different angles, using different parts of your tongue, pacing yourself, and making occasional eye contact.

- Use techniques like circles, sweeping, and the vacuum to enhance the cunnilingus experience.

- Know the signs to look for when she's enjoying the cunnilingus.

- Don't stop too soon.

Fundamental #13: Teach Her to Give You Great Head (so She Gets Addicted)

- Walk her through exactly how you want it, give her commands, and be dominant.

Fundamental #14: Consent and Protection

- Always get some form of consent before having sex with a girl.

- Always use protection to help prevent STDs and unwanted pregnancy.

Fundamental #15: 10 Amazing Sex Positions (and How to Use Them)

- Missionary with full contact

- Scissor doggy style

- Doggy style

- Lying flat doggy style

- Her on top

- Reverse cowgirl

- Edge-of-bed reverse cowgirl

- Mirror (or standing) doggy style

- Legs over shoulders

- Her on top while you're sitting on a chair

Fundamental #16: Dominance (The Right Way to Have Rough Sex)

- Give her commands instead of asking for permission.

- Pull her hair from the roots.

- Manhandle her to give her a little bit of pain with maximized psychological pleasure.

- Spank her.

- Come on her face, in her mouth, and/or on her tits.

Fundamental #17: Emotion

- Connect with her on an emotional level before sex. This will give you a foundation from which to make things more emotional and passionate during sex.

- Look into her eyes for ten to fifteen seconds while fucking her, and repeat this every couple of minutes.

- French kiss her to increase the level of intimacy.

- Moan and grunt to show her that you're enjoying the experience and that she's giving you pleasure.

Fundamental #18: The "Motion of the Ocean"

- Start with slow thrusts to set the pace and get into a good flow.

- Speed up your thrusts and then slow them back down to add variety and intensity to the sex.

- Use music as a guide and thrust to the tempo of the beat.

- Use your hips for more effective rhythmic thrusting.

- Occasionally thrust with your whole body to add more variety to the sex.

- Take a Latin dance class like salsa, as this will help you develop a natural sense of rhythm.

Fundamental #19: Dirty Talk

- Use possessive language to make it more personal and intimate.

- Tell her what you want.

- Say it like you mean it — don't let uncertainty creep into your voice.

- Tell her what you like to show her that she's giving you pleasure.

- Command her so she can let go and follow your lead.

Fundamental #20: Variety

- Alternate between different sex positions every seven to ten minutes.

- Have sex at different times of day.

- Have sex for different amounts of time.

- Use sex toys like blindfolds, handcuffs, and vibrators.

- Use varying levels of foreplay. Go for the full spectrum most of the time, but occasionally make it shorter or skip it altogether.

- Switch up locations between different apartments, rooms, and public places.

Fundamental #21: Orgasmic Anal Sex

- Get cleaned up beforehand so she feels comfortable with you going down there.

- Start slow so she can be both mentally and physically prepared before you penetrate her.

- Have lube ready to make penetration easier and less painful.

- Use the right positions so that she can orgasm.

- Thrust with slow, rhythmic movements.

Fundamental #22: Good Stamina and Breath Control

- Be in the moment so you can enjoy the experience without psyching yourself out.

- Control your breathing so you can pace yourself and avoid exhaustion.

- Switch to a less stimulating position if you feel like you're losing control, and switch to a less physically exhausting position if you feel like you're getting tired too quickly.

- Don't thrust constantly – slow down, rotate, and use other movements.

- Don't cycle through sexual techniques in your head.

- Hit the gym a few times a week to improve your physical stamina.

Fundamental #23: Get a "Main Girl"

- Your main girl basically provides a comfortable sexual environment for you to gradually improve in.

Fundamental #24: Practice Vulnerability

- Stay calm and composed, and be honest with the girl if you have a sexual mishap like coming too early or struggling to get an erection.

Fundamental #25: Get Harder Erections

- Go to the gym to improve your physique and boost your testosterone.

- Get better quality sleep so you have high energy

throughout the day and night.

- Avoid shitty foods that weigh you down and sap your energy.

- Drink less (or not at all) so that you're socially sharper and can perform well if you bring a girl home.

- Cut down on the porn/masturbation so that you don't desensitize yourself to physical intimacy.

Fundamental #26: Use These Tips to Last Longer

- Use less sensitive positons when you feel like you're about to come so that you can regain control before it's too late.

- Immerse yourself in the sexual experience and be in the moment instead of constantly thinking about when you're going to come.

- Stop and relax if you feel like the urge to come is getting overwhelming.

- Go multiple rounds. That way, if you come too quickly the first time, you can make it up to the girl in the next round.

- Use long-lasting condoms as a last resort – be careful, though, as they have numbing lubricants that dull pleasure and make sex a little less fun.

Fundamental #27: Show Her You Care

- *When you treat her well, it gives the girl positive emotions, improves your chances of seeing her again, and also increases her desire to please you.*

- *Avoid the common mistakes that most guys make, like asking her to leave immediately, acting weird, asking weird questions, etc.*

- *Show her you care by doing things like helping her clean up after sex, going for another round, and sending her a follow-up text the next day.*

Fundamental #28: Ask Her the Right Questions After Sex

- *What's a sexual fantasy you've always had?*

- *What's your favorite sex position?*

- *How rough do you like it?*

- *At what point did you realize you wanted to have sex with me?*

Your Next Step

There's no doubt in my mind that you're well on your way to becoming a sexual man, having mind-blowing sex, and giving women orgasm after orgasm!

But here's the thing...

The only way you can use these tips is if you attract women consistently and stay out of the friendzone.

Otherwise, you'll have all this great knowledge of sex but nobody to use it with!

That's why I'm giving you a FREE video series as an add-on to this book.

Get access now: *bit.ly/handbookcourse*

It features three in-depth videos, where I walk you through how to flirt with girls and avoid debilitating conversation mistakes that put you in the friendzone.

Inside you will learn:

- The five conversation mistakes that put you in the friendzone (and how to avoid them).

- My secret conversation framework for flirting with any girl.

- The "invisible trigger" that activates attraction in a woman's mind, often within seconds of meeting you.

- A simple way to overcome the three "dating roadblocks" that hold 99% of men back from meeting the women they truly want.

...and much, much more.

Get access now: ***bit.ly/handbookcourse***

Can You Do Me a Favor?

Thanks for checking out my book.

I'm confident you will master these fundamentals and dramatically improve your sex life if you follow what's written inside. But before you go, I have one small favor to ask...

Would you take 60 seconds and write a quick blurb about this book on Amazon?

Reviews are the best way for independent authors (like me) to get noticed, sell more books, and spread our message to as many people as possible. I also read every review and use the feedback to write future revisions – and future books, even.

Thank you – I really appreciate your support.

The Hook Up Handbook

About the Author

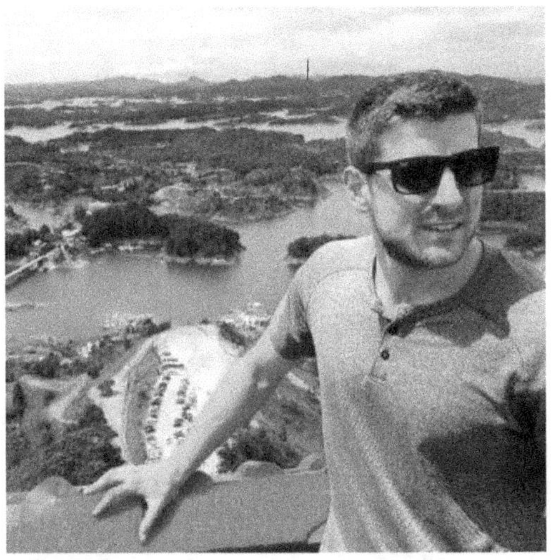

Dave Perrotta is a best-selling author, world traveler, and the founder of **PostGradCasanova.com** – a popular website for men who want to improve their dating lives, master conversation, have incredible sex, and become the best versions of themselves!

He's lived in 8 different countries in the past three years, become fluent in Spanish, met amazing women from many different cultures, and is constantly on some sort of crazy adventure.